Praise

"Rika Keck has pulled together valuable information in this book for patients with Lyme disease to navigate their personal nutritional needs and self-help treatments with ease. The Klinghardt Academy is in harmony with this amazing nutritional resource that embraces our 5 level healing model of spiritual, emotional, mind-body interventions. We highly recommend reading *Nourish, Heal, Thrive.*"

—**Debbie Floyd**, director, Klinghardt Academy

"This book is a grand tour of many key factors in chronic Lyme and provides readers a road map to wellness. I agree with the author that this book will 'guide, inspire, and empower' you on your healing path. By following the recommendations here, you will help your immune system regain its strength and greatly aid in your recovery."

—**Sunjya Schweig**, MD, CEO and codirector,
California Center for Functional Medicine

"This book is a *real* guide. Truly, the author has experienced all sides of chronic illness and has a desire to assist others in true healing and shortening their illness journey. I too have been the chronically ill patient who thought I would never heal, and I so wish I had this book then. Today, as a nutritionist with a focus on microbial illness and recovery, I will recommend this book to professionals and patients alike."

—**Karen Hubert**, Certified Natural Health Professional, North Carolina

"In this book, nutritional strategies and health supporting action steps are cornerstones for treating Lyme disease and related coinfections. The author, in addition, astutely enhances this mind-body approach by relating mold sensitivity; viral, fungal, and yeast challenges; fatigue; environmental toxicity; and emotional stress as integrating factors to the illness dynamics. Individuals who have been sick for some time will appreciate this information and physicians can consider it an excellent resource for treating their patients."

—**Morton M. Teich**, MD, past president, American Academy of Environmental Medicine; asthma and immunology fellow, American Academy of Allergy; committee-member, Adverse Reactions to Foods; instructor, Icahn Medical School of Mt. Sinai-Clinical

"For those with chronic Lyme and mold-related conditions, this is your comprehensive, wholesome, functional medicine-based book for healing your whole self. A must-have!"

—**Deanna Minich**, PhD, author of *Whole Detox*

"*Nourish Heal Thrive* is a game changer! Rika Keck reveals the hidden epidemic of Lyme disease that is sweeping across North America and spreading around the world. She takes us on a fascinating journey into this complex infection that robs so many of their health and vitality. Misunderstood and often ignored, people suffering from Lyme face an uphill battle for proper diagnosis and treatment. This functional and holistic approach provides nutritional, mind-body, gut, and detox strategies for fighting back against Lyme. This book will be a tremendous resource for health care professionals and the Lyme community for years to come."

—**Jonathan Galland**, JD, international best-selling coauthor of *The Allergy Solution*

"Living with Lyme disease can be devastating. Rika's book will both educate and empower you to follow a successful path to health."

—**Jeffrey A. Morrison**, MD, CNS, The Morrison Center, New York City

"Keck is the penultimate healer. She uniquely brings together her insights with those of other patients, doctors, and academics. *Nourish, Heal, Thrive* fills the knowledge gap for those whose lives have been directly or indirectly influenced by vector-borne infections. While the 'Lyme labyrinth' can be a daunting journey, Keck has soulfully cleared you a path to healing."

—**Alexander Rhinehardt**, DC, CNS, owner, Arizona Nutrition Center

"*Nourish, Heal, Thrive* provides a firm foundation for anyone willing to approach healing with an open mind and willing to consider the great amount each of us can do to heal, independent of—and in conjunction with—whatever your medical professional advises. It is a rare allopathic medical professional who has any knowledge of the measures Rika covers in this book. You will find here a true expansion of knowledge garnered from many sources—a first in client education. Rika's book outlines an area you *can* control, which can make all the mental and emotional difference as you deal with the often-devastating effects of environmental illness.

—**Linda Minarik**, ACE-certified fitness professional,
author of *Stretching with Ease*

Client Testimonials

"Rika's vast knowledge of chronic Lyme and how to support the mind and body via diet, supplements, herbs, and homeopathic methods has changed my life for the better. During our meetings, Rika helped me understand what is happening in my body and how I can take charge of my body and heal. She is not just an advisor; she is deeply committed to your well being as a friend would be, and that is how I regard her. When in doubt, I look through my notes and find an answer, which Rika has provided me with. And the chant about Drainage Tone, you'll have to ask her yourself. I can't sing her praises enough!"

—**Monika M.**, New York City

"I am feeling so much better than when I initially saw Rika. I feel like my Lyme is gone (for now at least), and I have been taking it easy at home and getting a lot of rest before I go back to school in two weeks. I am trying to watch my diet and sleeping habits and nutrient and supplement intake."

—**Abi**, New Jersey

"Rika is the first person to truly get to the bottom of my digestive issues. I've finally found some relief for the first time in three years because she hasn't given up. She's offered continuous advice and support by suggesting various supplements or tests. Rika has been a professional advisor but also a friend who really cares about my health."

—**Arrington R.**, Washington DC

"I have experienced digestive troubles since I was twelve years of age. I've tried the macrobiotic, vegan, and vegetarian diets, but they also affected my hormones badly and they did not help me feel any better. At that time, my doctor said I had IBS. I continued having symptoms such as constipation, diarrhea, hemorrhoid pain, and bloating. I was so glad when I started working with Rika. After our consultation we started on elimination of high FODMAP foods and high histamine foods as I was experiencing SIBO-associated symptoms. I also stopped taking my probiotics that contained inulin. After a short while of food eliminations, I felt so much better! No more constipation and diarrhea! My hemorrhoid pain decreased, and I was able to have bowl movements with no pain. We then added proteolytic enzymes that made me feel a lot better, and Rika suggested that I add additional red root for lymphatic drainage. At present, I am able to tolerate high FODMAP foods and I experience no more pain when having bowl movements. When I went to see my gastroenterologist, I mentioned that I was consulting with a functionally minded nutritional health coach. He remarked, 'Your nutritionist must be really smart for having you eliminate high FODMAP foods!'"

—**By Angela**, New Jersey

"My upstate Lyme-treating doctor and nurse practitioner recommended Rika to me. I was told that Rika works with complex digestive cases regarding nutrition, especially within the scenario of chronic Lyme. I was misdiagnosed for quite some time, and it has been eighteen years since I first became sick with Lyme.

In 2014, my ENT diagnosed me with esophageal reflux and he prescribed acid blockers. They seemed to work, and my voice began to sound clear again. But, after sixty days, I suffered a horrible rebound and ended up seeing two nutrition specialists, neither of whom helped. I also saw two GI doctors. I did not want more medications, and I was pretty sure that any additional medication would create a problem. Finally a gastroenterologist diagnosed me with SIBO.

SIBO wrecked my voice. Vocal hoarseness made it impossible for me to sing or even hum for over three years. At one point, my speaking voice became so croaky and distorted that is was unrecognizable to family and friends over the phone. The vocal problems were in addition to acute abdominal pain, never-ending burping and gas, and sleep disruption.

I was desperate to find a protocol that would work for me. When Rika and I started working, I could hardly hum three tones. Everything else was gone. Being unable to sing was a great loss to me. I am now in my fifth month with the SIBO diet, and I find my voice returning. I now have eight notes!

As tough as the SIBO diet is—and it is toug—it gets results. Rika takes her time to explain the different stages required, especially while also not wanting to stir up a herx. After only three weeks of the diet, the pain lessened. The giant frog burps began to calm down. The improvement in sleep has improved the quality of my life. I've had some setbacks along the way, but the improvement in my voice is enough to keep me going. Many people have remarked how much better I sound, and I have been able to gain weight. That, plus generous servings of nut butters. (After all, I am low weight.)

I hope to spread this information to other people who are suffering and not getting anywhere with standard medical treatment. If someone is willing to commit to the food regimen, they will see improvement. I am grateful that I contacted Rika, and we are still working together. Months, or even a year, of food restrictions is better than many years of pain and physical limitation."

—**Linda H.**, Upstate New York

"Good news: My menstrual period began today. Feel so happy and relaxed; I can't even tell you how glad I am today!!! This is all Rika's great work! Thank God I met her!"

—**Karina**, New York City

"Thank you very much, Rika. After eight years of searching and dozen of doctors, I feel that finally someone who understands my child's symptoms and is able to help me fight Lyme disease and its complications. Since working with Rika, I began to hope that my daughter can heal and have a happy childhood. We changed the diet, and I learned ways to improve her daily life—methods and supplements to support her weaken body and to improve her immune system. I know that this is a long, long road, but I feel that now we can hope."

—**Relly Nedelcu**

"I had a sizeable decrease in burping and gas over the months that I've been following the regimen Rika laid out for me. My sleep has improved, and with better sleep I've experienced a reduction in joint pain. Last month, I actually had a few, maybe three, days during the month when I woke up clear-headed, had energy, and was able to get through the day of tasks without needing to lie down. This is a very big deal. Very. I call these 'normal days' because they're the kind normal (i.e., not sick) people have."

—L. H.

. . . . .

You never know how
strong you are
until being strong
is your only choice.

—UNKNOWN

. . . . .

RIKA KECK

ACN, CMTA, FDN-P

NOURISH

HEAL

THRIVE

A COMPREHENSIVE & HOLISTIC APPROACH
TO LIVING WITH LYME DISEASE

RIVER GROVE
BOOKS

This book is intended for informational purposes and as a reference volume only. It is not intended as a medical manual and/or self-diagnosis of disease. The information given here is designed to help you make informed decisions about your health. It is not intended as a substitute for any treatment that may have been prescribed by your doctor. If you suspect that you have a medical problem, you should seek competent medical help and avoid self-treatment, especially when existing medical problems are already present. You should neither begin a new health regimen without first consulting a medical professional, nor stop or change any prescribed treatment protocols. The author and publisher specifically disclaim any liability, loss, or risk, personal or otherwise, which is incurred as a consequence, directly or indirectly, of the use and application of any contents of this book. Individuals are solely responsible for their own health-care decisions. The author and publisher specifically disclaim any liability for any adverse reaction or event, loss, or risk, personal or otherwise, which is incurred as a consequence, directly or indirectly, of the use and application of any contents of this book. Potential sources of information including websites, organizations, and supplements are for general information only, and it does not mean that the author agrees or endorses all health claims made by these sites, organizations, and products companies.

Published by River Grove Books
Austin, TX
www.rivergrovebooks.com

Distributed by River Grove Books

Design and composition by Greenleaf Book Group
Cover design by Greenleaf Book Group
Cover images: ©iStockphoto/4kodiak

Cataloging-in-Publication data is available.

Print ISBN: 978-1-63299-099-0

eBook ISBN: 978-1-63299-100-3

First Edition

For Mom

You believed in me; this is for you.

To my husband and my families

You have stood continuously by my side; thank you.

To the reader

May this book shine a guiding light on your courageous path towards wellness. You are the inspiration and motivation for this book.

In gratitude to those who have stood by my side at all times, encouraged me, and helped make this book possible.

Thank you, Ronald Lauder.

Table of Contents

Foreword

Rika Keck has written a beautiful and essential text for the chronic Lyme patient. Over the last ten years, I have treated nearly four thousand patients with Lyme disease, and, as time has gone on, our model for treatment has changed. Beginning with more traditional antibiotics many years ago, today I prescribe very few antibiotics. Instead, I use mostly natural, integrative therapies to recover patients from the most formidable states of health. Patients with no quality of life to speak of come to our clinic and, hopefully, with love, care, and targeted protocols, are able to regain their lives.

The journey has humbled me as a practitioner and made me acutely aware of the intense suffering these patients experience. This task in my hands has brought me to a higher level of spiritual self-awareness in order to be strong and able to impart the love and light that these patients desperately need.

Rika's beautiful text summarizes the basic philosophy that so many of us identify with in the field. It underscores the power of kindness, love, and non-judgment on the road to recovery and emphasizes the importance of using the body's God-given pathways of healing and detoxification in order to support this journey. It is an essential text for anyone that is suffering from chronic disease. I am so moved by her work that I will make it a must read for all of my patients.

Just as every oyster bears a pearl, so too is the journey back from chronic illness. The demanding spiritual growth that is necessary to fully recover from chronic Lyme disease often forces my patients to ultimately lead an improved, more fulfilled, and productive life after recovery than before. I can only imagine that with the assistance of this book, the path will come more easily now.

With respect and gratitude,

Kristine Gedroic, MD,
Diplomate of the American Board of Medical Acupuncture and the American Board of Integrative Medicine, the Gedroic Center for Integrative Medicine in Morristown, New Jersey

Preface

Writing this book is certainly a far cry from my days as a professional ballet dancer in South Africa. Never during my *Swan Lake* years would I have considered the path I have taken. It was not until after I survived a terrible car accident that kept me in bed for many weeks, followed by a slow rehab, that I knew I had a purpose—but I did not know what it was at that time. Today, I do know what it is: to teach, guide, inspire, and empower.

Since moving to New York City in 2001, I have attended many conferences on clinical nutrition, women's wellness, chronic disease and inflammation, functional and environmental medicine, supporting patients with cancer, and chronic Lyme disease. I have certainly seen many airports and conference rooms—and hotel gyms, as exercise has always been important to me.

One of my earliest inspirations in regards to studies in chronic Lyme and persistent infections was a conference featuring Dr. Dietrich Klinghardt. Because I grew up in South Africa in a German household, I appreciated his German accent and broad way of thinking. I learned firsthand about various medical, botanical, and energetic interventions, as well as healing with Family Constellations, a therapy addressing multigenerational systemic dynamics. The complexities of Lyme disease propelled me into ongoing studies over the past ten years. More recently, in 2016, I was thrilled to attend Dr. Klinghardt's lectures at The Forum of Integrative Medicine Conference.

I have had many terrific teachers over the years, and I am grateful for all I have learned from them. The work of Dr. Kristine Gedroic; herbalists Susan McAmish, Lee Carol, and Kerry Bone; Dr. Anne Corson; Dr. Stuart White; Dr.

Richard Horowitz; Dr. Jeffrey Bland; Dr. Alex Vasquez; Dr. Alan McDonald; and Dr. Patricia Kane have all influenced my life and practice. They are not afraid to push the boundaries of conventional medical thinking, which is currently based on pathology and symptom suppression. Learning from forward-thinking professionals has certainly put me at odds with allopathic thinking when it comes to chronic illnesses. Just recently, I returned from the American Academy of Environmental Medicine conference that was dedicated to the impact of environmental toxicity on mitochondrial dysfunction, a real concern in the toxic world we live in today.

It is my belief that we are whole beings and must be addressed from a mind-body perspective. From my own experiences, I know that emotional burdens play a large role in physical disease. Thus, I became immersed in mind-body work, studying Reiki, medical intuition, and Psych-K, all of which address subconscious belief patterns.

It was my commitment to holistic health that inspired me to create NY Integrated Health, LLC, in 2006. At the time, I was a top-notch New York City physical trainer, working with knee replacements and rotator cuff issues, and teaching group fitness classes in midtown Manhattan. Meanwhile, my head was stirring with the latest information I had learned at conferences and webinars.

With an ambitious, curious, and problem-solving predisposition, I was not satisfied with addressing the physical body and physiology in the context of conventional medicine. I was interested in *why* symptoms occurred and the investigative approach of root-cause resolution.

During my time as an educator, I was the host of a twelve-week online radio program called *Dynamo Lunch Radio*. I interviewed integrative New York City physicians, a farm-to-table restaurateur, functional psychiatrists, a women's wellness pelvic therapist, a holistic dentist, and more. I very much enjoyed these shows that helped me when I was going through a very difficult time.

While amassing multiple certifications—such as Functional Diagnostic Nutrition Practitioner, Certified Metabolic Typing Advisor, Holistic Lifestyle Coach, and Reiki One and Two—and attending medical conferences across the United States, I became convinced that I could best be of service as a holistic practitioner and health advocate for individuals who were suffering from chronic illness, especially Lyme. Many had fallen through the cracks of conventional medicine.

My continuous studies opened my eyes to how I could support my clients from a personalized nutritional, holistic, and functional paradigm. All along, I was staying abreast of cutting-edge information regarding chronic Lyme, vector-borne infections, biotoxins, and environmental medicine. In the meantime, I have been honored to collaborate with various medical professionals, including Lyme-literate medical doctors.

Through the years, I have dealt with my own health challenges, including multiple skin cancer surgeries, physical injuries, and family illness. I was also faced with the devastating and very sudden loss of my mom in 2014.

While supporting clients with chronic Lyme from a nutritional and clinical perspective (not treating the disease), I felt compelled to write this comprehensive book. It is not just about the illness; it is about the terrain. Many symptoms can be caused by vector-borne infections, yet our daily nutritional and lifestyle choices, plus environmental toxin exposures, can harm and provoke the body too. I have witnessed grateful clients who have more energy, can tolerate more foods, and have become more empowered through the process of learning how they can use food to help themselves heal. This has given renewed hope and joy to lives that were involved in an ongoing struggle for many years.

My clients tell me, "You get it."

And to me, there is no higher compliment.

Introduction

This book is written especially for sufferers of chronic Lyme sickness. You have probably already been on a difficult journey with many twists and turns over the past months, and possibly many years. I welcome you to share the information in this book with those around you who might not be aware of the challenges associated with your current illness. This book is also for those who have recovered after prolonged antibiotic or herbal treatment and who are seeking to improve their nutrition and whole-body wellness following years of sickness. There are always healing opportunities that can fortify us on our individual wellness journey.

First came the infection, often from a tick bite. Maybe you saw the tick that infected you, developed a rash and flu-like symptoms, and, hopefully, got prompt treatment. Or maybe you did not know you had been bitten. You might never have had the classic bull's eye rash (Erythema Migrans) associated with Lyme disease. Fewer than fifty percent of individuals recall seeing a rash, which can take many different shapes and forms.

Transfer from the saliva of a tick can happen in less than twenty-four hours. It is a myth that this can only occur after twenty-four to forty-eight hours, and there is sufficient data to support faster transmission times.[1] My husband was infected by a tick in less than three hours. Not all ticks carry infectious agents, but many of them do. Without medical or other antimicrobial intervention within the first weeks, it increases the likelihood of insidious and severe sickness over many years.

When the tick attaches to the host, it burrows its barbed mouthparts into the body, injecting substances similar to an anesthetic and antihistamine. As a result, you do not feel the tick latch on, and it begins to feed. The tick also releases enzymes and an anticlotting substance. Clotting protects the body from external infectious assaults or injuries, so the injected substance deactivates the immune system, keeping it from responding appropriately to the invasion.

Dismantling these protective gatekeepers allows for the easy transfer of Lyme spirochetes, worms (nematodes) containing spirochetes, parasites, toxins, and other infectious agents, from the tick to the host. If undisturbed, the tick will burrow into the skin and feed on the host's blood for several days, growing in size and releasing infectious agents into the body. Once fully satiated and engorged, the tick will release and fall off. The longer it stays attached, the more risk there is for harmful transmission.

Without appropriate therapeutic intervention, the more potential there is for insidious and mysterious sicknesses. Once inside the body, Lyme spirochetes choose transportation highways and hiding places outside the bloodstream, where the immune system cannot get to them easily. Lyme's infectious agents can be in spirochete (corkscrew), granular, round ball, and cyst forms.[2] The bacteria change shape as needed to avoid detection in the host, and they prefer round forms to evade antibiotic therapy. They effectively use the lymphatic system and the peripheral nervous system for their transportation network. Sanctuaries can include the brain, inside the eyeball and joints that are rich in hyaluronic acid, and heart tissue. The infection seeks ways to avoid detection and ensure its survival.

But maybe you were not infected by a tick . . .

Many people do not know that transfer of infectious bacteria, toxins, and parasites can also occur from mosquito, flea, sandfly, bed bug, or spider bites; excrement from fleas on beloved pets; perhaps semen and vaginal fluids during sexual activities; a scratch from your cat or dog; raw milk; breast milk; saliva; pregnancy; and blood transfusions. Blacklegged ticks are not the only culprits. Because transmission is possible via various vectors, we now refer to these infections as *vector-borne infections*.

The guidelines for an acute infection are set by the Centers for Disease

Control and Prevention (CDC). If clinical symptoms such as a skin rash, severe headaches, or facial palsy are present, treatment consists of two to four weeks of 100 to 200 mg of oral doxycycline, amoxicillin, or cefuroxime axetil (once or twice per day). This is standard antibiotic treatment for Lyme, or *borreliosis*. In severe cardiovascular and neurologic conditions, acute IV treatment with penicillin and ceftriaxone is advocated.[3]

However, the standard dose and duration of antibiotic treatment is often not enough to eliminate the infection. In addition, various coinfections that are transmitted simultaneously do not respond to standard antibiotic treatment. This contributes to the development of a complex chronic illness, and symptoms can occur over the next weeks and months, or many years later.

Currently, there is no evidence that infectious microbes are eliminated or that an individual is cured after commercial short-term (two to four week) antibiotic treatment. According to the International Lyme and Disease Society (ILADS) website, forty percent of infected individuals continue to have chronic health problems after initial short-term antibiotic treatment.

Lyme is a modern-day epidemic with multiple strains and various mutations that are unique to specific regions in the world. The disease is grossly misunderstood and misdiagnosed. Politics are at play within the scientific and medical community, insurance companies, and government agencies.

According to the CDC, roughly 300,000 cases of Lyme disease are diagnosed in the United States each year. But Lyme and other vector-borne infections are grossly underreported as testing is unreliable. In North America, *Borrelia burgdorferi* is prevalent; however, in Europe, Asia, and Russia, more diverse strains are common, including *Borrelia garinii*, *Borrelia miyamotoi* with relapsing fever, and *Borrelia afzelii*. It is possible to be coinfected with two different strains of *Borrelia*.[4] If you know where you were infected, returning to that location for specific strain testing is ideal.

Unfortunately for those suffering from chronic Lyme, according to the CDC and the Infectious Disease Society of America (IDSA), which receives funding from the CDC, chronic Lyme disease does not exist. Instead, the CDC gives the multisystemic illness a vague label: *Post-Treatment Lyme Disease Syndrome*.

In the United States, the CDC's two-tiered testing guidelines are used for

Lyme disease. Testing is based on a single strain of a spirochete, called *B. burg-dorferi*, from the gut of a tick. Yet there are over a hundred different known strains of *B. burgdorferi* in the United States and hundreds of different strains abroad. These two-tiered tests do not check for various coinfections that are often transmitted with the Lyme infection. False or negative results are not uncommon despite presence of active infections and symptoms of sickness.

Infections suppress the immune system and lower our body temperature because they like to operate in a cooler environment. With a compromised immune system, we are more susceptible to airborne viral infections, such as malaria and the West Nile and Zika viruses, or the reactivation of latent herpes viruses inside the body. Combinations of infectious disease and viral activity are key factors in multisystemic illnesses, and they can be deadly.

There are many coinfections that can be layered with *Borrelia*, which has many different strains. Prevalent coinfections in North America include various strains of *Babesia* (babesiosis), *Ehrlichia* (ehrlichiosis), *Bartonella henselae* (also known as cat scratch fever), *Rickettsia rickettsii* (Rocky Mountain spotted fever), and Southern tick-associated rash illness (STARI). Infections such as *Bartonella* and *Babesia* can exist inside cells and in the fluid surrounding cells (also known as the *extracellular matrix*), where Lyme spirochetes are active. In addition, there are microorganisms that contribute to other tenacious infections, such as *Myco-plasma, Anaplasma, Chlamydia pneumoniae*, and the Powassan virus, which is related to the mosquito-borne West Nile virus (now reported in forty-eight states in this country[5]). Often other dormant viral infections become activated, such as Epstein-Barr virus, cytomegalovirus, herpes simplex virus 1 and 2, and more. It is not just the Lyme infection that makes us sick, but rather the overlapping of multiple infections and ongoing inflammation.

Often, patients are dismissed by their doctors, who believe their symptoms must be psychosomatic, and are sent to psychiatrists. Children and adults are often misdiagnosed with mental illnesses without consideration of Lyme or other stealth infections.[6] Lyme and *Bartonella* coinfections, plus the latent impact of strep infections in the brain, as seen in pediatric autoimmune neuropsychiatric disorders associated with streptococcal infections (PANDAS), have been known to cause cardiovascular, psychiatric, and behavioral problems in babies and children.[7] This is not considered in conventional psychiatry, pediatric care, or cardiology. However, it is encouraging that organizations such as PANDAS Network provide scientific research and education into the medical arena.

More than a million people are infected with vector-borne illnesses, many of whom do not know it. Lyme is known as *The Great Imitator*. Hidden coinfections and viruses masquerade with mysterious symptoms that mimic other diseases and illnesses. This results in autoimmune, cardiovascular, neurological, digestive, arthritic, and psychiatric symptoms that are often misdiagnosed. Various government agencies, insurance companies, and physicians do not believe that Lyme disease causes such illnesses. Even if tests are inconclusive, the so-called *mysterious symptoms* from Lyme and other associated infections are not imagined by sick individuals. Symptoms are very real, and they affect those suffering from chronic Lyme every single day and night.

Absence of proof is not proof of absence: Infections can remain dormant for many years and then appear at a later stage in life when the immune system is compromised or after a very stressful event or trauma. When this occurs, many individuals are often misdiagnosed as having fibromyalgia, chronic fatigue syndrome, heart arrhythmia, irritable bowel syndrome, autism, interstitial cystitis, depression, or a degenerative neurological disease such as multiple sclerosis, Alzheimer's, dementia, or Parkinson's disease.

Many who have been on this long road of undiagnosed or misdiagnosed illnesses end up with multiple prescriptions for anxiety and mood disorders, addictive analgesics, and sleeping medications; yet they are medically ill with multiple infections and biotoxins. It is understandable if a sense of hopelessness emerges. All this can make you feel overwhelmed, chronically fatigued, and depressed because you are unable to function in your daily life, and you feel you are sliding into a dark abyss.

You are not alone.

One patient suffering from chronic Lyme expressed that she felt she was becoming a shadow of herself and that she was slowly dying. Another client is unable to work because of physical disabilities in her hands and arms. She was misdiagnosed with chronic fatigue syndrome, but she knew something else was going on. Disrupted sleep patterns, chronic fatigue, and cognitive dysfunction are common symptoms with persistent Lyme and coinfections. With Lyme disease and coinfections, many suffer from major digestive troubles after years of analgesics, antibiotics, and acid-blocking medication. Others end up in wheelchairs because they lose the use of their legs. The severe debilitation that can accompany these persistent infections can result in paralysis; spasticity of limbs, jaw, and face; and death. Some individuals even contemplate suicide out of sheer desperation, exhausted from the endless struggles, insomnia, and ongoing pain.

Those who are finally diagnosed and choose a pharmaceutical or integrative approach embark on a path of multiple rotations of various antibiotics and antimicrobial medications that affect their energy, digestion, mood, gut health, and ability to think clearly. As the body kills bacteria and parasites, it can cause some to feel even sicker during treatment. Sometimes the reaction to medicines and pain from migraines, seizures, and muscle spasms can lead to an emergency room visit, which is further complicated by the belief of most attending medical professionals that chronic Lyme does not exist.

Many people do not understand how difficult it can be just to get out of bed to take a shower or to go grocery shopping when ongoing fatigue and pain from infections engulf the body. Sometimes, memory is so affected that those suffering do not remember the way back home from the doctor. Many don't understand how difficult it can be for someone who is ill and struggling with cognition to focus at work with terrible headaches, if one is able to work at all. Individuals drop out of school, endure breakups, divorce, rejection from family members, loss of a job, and financial ruin.

Financing complex treatment or travel to doctors in other states is also a challenge. The bills for Lyme-literate medical doctors, medications, lab tests, IV infusions, and supplements can be astronomical. Arguments on the telephone with the insurance companies regarding possible longer-term coverage of antibiotics or other medical tests are common. These frustrations siphon energy that those with chronic Lyme do not have.

Is everyone with persistent Lyme and coinfections this ill? No, but many are. Many sufferers are able to recover after prolonged antibiotic treatment or after alternative treatments. Those who opt for a nonpharmaceutical approach often have to defend that decision against strong opposition from doctors and loved ones. Sadly, there are also individuals who are diagnosed very late, and they succumb to the disease after years of suffering.

It is my intention to present a neutral perspective regarding treatment options; the choice is yours to make. Financial concerns always come into play, and they affect any treatment choice. Not everyone with Lyme wants, can afford, or tolerates antibiotic treatment, which can go on for years. Many chose another path, healing themselves using nutrition, alternative botanical protocols, and complementary treatments. Others integrate a pharmaceutical, herbal, and homeopathic approach. Every case is different.

This book is also intended as a patient education resource for allopathic and Lyme-literate physicians, because there is often limited time in a consultation to cover the comprehensive subject of nutritional self-help. It provides nutritional and functional information that complements every therapeutic protocol. No matter what treatment is chosen, nutrition, lifestyle, lowering of stress, and avoiding toxic environmental exposures must be integrated in a healing strategy.

Vector-borne infections and Lyme disease are a real challenge in the world today. Testing is not foolproof, prolonged medical treatment is costly, and politics within government agencies, insurance companies, and the medical and scientific communities prevent effective and large-scale progress from being made.

Even within the Lyme-literate medical community, opinions regarding prolonged antibiotic use and alternative therapeutic treatment protocols vary. Alternative health practitioners who work in this arena criticize the heavy emphasis on antibiotic treatment and the infection. Their belief is that the disease has consequences beyond the infection itself, and it is vital to emphasize the constitution of the person as a whole and not just focus on killing the pathogens.

I applaud the physicians, scientists, institutions, and foundations involved in research—in particular ILADS, which takes on government policies and strives to increase funding, education, and awareness of the debilitating effects of these chronic infections. Lyme disease organizations around the world strongly push for research and the need for specialized testing to ensure an early diagnosis, with an emphasis on patient-centered care for restoration of health and quality of life.

. . . .

Wrapping Up

As a holistic practitioner, I am aware that many individuals choose not to use long-term antibiotics. Prolonged use of antibiotics affects biological systems of the body, including our gut microbiome. The good news is that there are many alternative healing options. Some physicians use only nutritional and herbal approaches; others might pulse, integrating short-term IV antibiotics to lower the initial microbial load or during a flare-up; others choose long-term IV antibiotics or oral medications.

Living with chronic infections is complex, but remember what Louis Pasteur recanted on his deathbed: "Bernard was right; the pathogen is nothing; the terrain is everything." In order to achieve a renewed sense of wellness when living with vector-borne infections, we must focus on the whole person, with an emphasis on nutrition, lifestyle, detoxification, hidden gut challenges, toxic loads, heavy metals, and underlying viral infections that suppress the immune system.

All of these components are important in the labyrinth of Lyme-related infections. My intention is not to tell you how to treat or cure your chronic Lyme and the coinfections. Instead, this book is geared toward building resilience so you can tolerate your medical and alternative therapeutic protocols for your sickness, so you may experience better days, more energy, and renewed hope in your life. I encourage you to trust your instincts and modify the general information in this book according to your unique needs.

Chapter One

Nourish, Heal, Thrive

To improve our resilience in regards to chronic infections, we must place great emphasis on nourishment, beginning with the foods we eat. Consider this book a starting point for your specific dietary needs and a trusted self-help guide that reveals how foods can heal or harm you. No, it is not about recipes and shakes; it is about exploring foods that are ideal—or not—for you today. I know that your daily dietary needs and your ability to tolerate foods can fluctuate with symptom flare-ups and side effects from medications, so you need to customize your daily choices to what you can tolerate at a certain time.

When you are feeling nauseous from medications and are herxing, you might only be able to tolerate a few sips of chicken soup or a bowl of oatmeal. (Herxing is named after Adolf Jarish and Karl Herxheimer. It describes a systemic inflammatory reaction after antimicrobial treatment is introduced and the body is not able to clear the die-off toxins.) Your body knows best.

After prolonged illness with antibiotic treatment and other medications, many people suffer from digestive dysfunction, which affects their resilience and ability to thrive. Treating infections without addressing the individual's unique milieu will not bring desired results. Consider the following:

- Prolonged stress of any kind alters your gut terrain, inflames the body, and increases toxicity. This plays an important role in your ability to heal and flourish after years of illness.
- How efficiently you eliminate toxins plays an important part in your ability to become well.

- Our gut houses up to seventy percent of the immune system; thus, our gut terrain is a major component of any personalized healing strategy.

This book goes into great detail regarding optimal food options and overall digestive wellness strategies. The collateral damage from long-term use of oral antibiotics and other medications is debilitating for the gut, because they alter the flora diversity and internal regulation between different microbial species.

Our gut health plays an important role in our energy, mood, and resilience; we must keep that in mind, especially because some infections, such as Lyme and *Bartonella*, can directly target the gut, making us feel depressed and anxious. Digestive function is compromised when chronic infections are present, and this raises various questions, including—

- Can healthy foods give you a headache?
- How does your gut flora affect your food sensitivities?
- Are you eating the right fats and oils that lower inflammation?
- How does your stomach lining affect your chronic joint pain?
- What role does your gallbladder play in your inability to tolerate healthy fats?

Many have sought out nutritional counseling in the past in an attempt to alleviate digestive troubles and extreme energy slumps while also treating their Lyme infections. However, when it comes to secondary gut infections, such as *Blastocystis hominis*, *Cryptosporidium*, small intestinal bacterial overgrowth (SIBO), and *Giardia*, nutritional modifications without targeted antimicrobial interventions will not be effective. Advanced gut testing from specialized labs is helpful in ruling out hidden infections in the digestive tract. This is all part of the Lyme labyrinth.

When it comes to what foods are best for you, consider that specific influences, including your ancestral traits, environment, financial means, stress levels, gut health, and food preparation all matter. A question I often hear from my clients is, "What foods can I eat?" I wrote this book to help you answer this question. I am sure you know that what you eat affects your digestive symptoms, but how do you choose which diet is right for you when there are so many to choose from? It can be very confusing.

The environment and food availability have changed tremendously in the last hundred years. We are able to preserve, ship, and transport foods around the globe and are now eating foods that do not correspond to our immediate environment and climate. If you are living in a cold climate, you want to eat warming foods, such as stewed meats or braised vegetables; compare this to eating cooling foods like salads or watermelon, which are ideal in the summer or when living in a tropical climate. Food availability during different seasons is important because locally grown, seasonal foods support our body's needs in our specific climate. It is time to see the big picture—your own unique dietary picture within your immediate environment.

Maybe you are hoping to find out what the perfect diet is for dealing with the collateral damage from Lyme infections. If I said this book will provide you with all the answers, I would be untruthful.

There is no such thing as a perfect diet. We are all different.

Just as we each have a different shoe size, we each have a different biochemical makeup. Yes, many of us wear a size eight shoe, but there are many variances to consider. For example, how wide does the shoe need to be to accommodate a bunion, a longer second toe, or a wider foot? What color or style of the size eight shoe do you prefer? With persistent chronic Lyme infections, you need a fortified and resilient shoe that fits your unique foot—and one that can handle any terrain. Your dietary needs are unique, and they must be seen in context with your ability to digest foods at the present time. With your health challenges, you need a customized nutritional approach that fortifies and energizes your body and mind so you can get back into a life of fulfillment and productivity.

Your body knows what it needs to help you get better; it is best to closely assess how you feel when you eat foods after each meal. Some individuals respond better to a diet high in protein and healthy fats, and others feel ill when eating a lot of fatty foods, even if the fats are healthy. If you are salivating for a lamb chop, that is your body talking. If you dislike dark meats and prefer to eat a plate of vegetables, that is also your body talking. Listen to it. (The Healthexcel System of Metabolic Typing can be very helpful in fine-tuning your dietary needs.) Common examples of how our dietary needs change as our bodies change include a pregnant woman who may be craving foods she did not care for prior to pregnancy; or when a woman experiences chocolate cravings before menstruation, and then the craving dissipates after a few days; or when you are not feeling well, chicken soup is welcome, but a Cobb salad is not. Thus, a generalized approach does not work, even though it certainly would be easier if there was a one-size-fits-all diet for individuals dealing with persistent Lyme and toxic mold illness.

Some foods may not agree with you. With a sluggish gallbladder, which often occurs with chronic infections and various medications, fat digestion can be a challenge; yet we need a variety of fatty acids to protect our brain, to lower inflammation, to support our hormones, and to help us function. Other foods might cause you to experience bloating or gas. There are various possible reasons for this, and I will address many of them in this book. Respecting your unique nutritional needs is key.

Ultimately, it is not about the food, it is about how your unique biochemistry responds to the foods you eat. You might already be following a specific dietary path and feel some improvement but have reached a plateau. The information in this book can take you to the next level, or it might present you with an angle you had not considered before—especially when it comes to your nutrient absorption, gut flora health, and blood sugar balance. And if no one has ever mentioned gut repair, mitochondrial function, membrane wellness, butyrate, or glutathione to you, you will know all about it by the time you finish reading this book.

This book is not about a specific diet. Instead, it is about creating your own eating plan that works for you and makes you feel better by lowering inflammation, giving you energy, decreasing bloating, preventing unwanted weight gain, and supporting your gut restoration.

You can choose any dietary approach (and there are so many), yet none of them will be effective if you do not consider the important role of digestion, absorption, and elimination. All must be optimized, especially when dealing with multiple symptoms from Lyme-related infections. I recommend making gut healing part of your daily nourishing program because it plays a very important role in your long-term ability to thrive. Each step of the digestive process matters, and when it functions correctly, you will be able to eat a wide variety of foods without indigestion, bloating, or blood sugar crashes.

By following the action steps provided in this book, you will nourish your depleted body and heal your gut by—

- Exploring optimal food choices that you can tolerate
- Accessing an insider's perspective of why you may not be able to tolerate certain foods
- Learning about the important fats and oils that lower inflammation
- Optimizing food preparation for your individual challenges
- Lowering your stress
- Implementing helpful tips to improve the function and health of your digestive tract
- Increasing your energy by supporting your brain and adrenals
- Supporting blood sugar balance with food choices
- Optimizing your ability to detox, so you can lower the accumulated toxic burden in the body
- Moving on a daily basis, choosing options that make you feel better and think better
- Resetting the mind (Instead of being defined as a chronic Lyme patient, reestablish your identity as a creative, gifted, and spiritual being who is on a human journey.)

My philosophy is a positive approach—focus on the foods you can eat, rather than focusing on what not to eat (that only reinforces sabotage and cravings). Do not try to be perfect; that is impossible and will only create added stress. However, elimination of inflammatory food triggers such as refined sugar, processed foods that are high in sodium, gluten, yeast-containing foods, partially hydrogenated vegetable oils, and soy is necessary if you want to become well.

Multiple food intolerances and hidden infections increase inflammation, drain your hormones, affect your fertility and bone health, and cause fatigue. There are informative guidelines and nutritional action steps in this book to help you navigate your dietary conundrum. Some action steps may be familiar to you, and some may not. Implementing these over time will help your body's ability to deal with infections as your energy increases.

Throughout the book, I mention nutritional, herbal, and homeopathic supplementation that complement customized dietary strategies, but know that I believe in a foundational food-first approach. This book will give general information regarding supplements that can assist you on your dietary path, but you must discuss your unique situation with your physician before starting *any* supplementation.

Everyone has challenges when living with Lyme, and everyone responds differently to different foods. As such, this book is created as a general guide, not as a nutritional prescription. Take your time; take it page by page. I hope that you will find it helpful and that it will make your life better. I invite you to start on the path to support your overall wellness.

When it comes to what you eat, spending time shopping and on food preparation will take work and energy. A sometimes complex schedule of medications and supplements is an additional challenge, especially when you are feeling tired. So think about what you can you do to add energy into every day. Rest periods? Meditation? Planning adequate rest helps to lower your stress, and you will have more stamina for self-care during the day. Rather than thinking of this as work, why not consider taking care of yourself as part of a nourishing lifestyle?

. . . .

Wrapping Up

Become mindful of the foods you choose to eat: They can help heal you. When you hold a bunch of celery or kale in your hand, is it not a marvel, this gift nature gives us? When making broth from bones, is it not a gift that the animal kingdom gives us? Maintaining a sense of gratitude in adversity is helpful during tough times; it reconnects us to healing and hope.

Nourishment from loving relationships will increase your resilience in the face of the tough reality that you deal with every day that not many understand. I will be frank; living with Lyme, coinfections, and mold illness can be a tough, lonely, expensive, and overwhelming road. Navigating daily life with a lack of stamina can be a difficult process (especially if you are living alone).

By connecting with Mother Nature and your inner spiritual being, you can open up channels of hope and healing that will support your immune system, lift your mood, and reduce your hormonal stress. Taking care of yourself also includes appropriate daily movement. Do what you can, go slow, and take appropriate rest afterward. Movement supports flow of your lymphatic and digestive systems and energizes the mind and body.

We have to nourish as a whole from a mind-body perspective. This takes mindfulness, careful planning, and patience; it is a slow process, and it takes practice. Lowering your stress with daily biofeedback techniques, deep breathing exercises, or meditation will greatly assist you in getting back into a life that is not defined by Lyme-related infections, chronic fatigue, and hopelessness.

It is very important to be kind to yourself. Surround yourself with supportive family, friends, and colleagues who understand your daily challenges without judgments. Emotional nourishment also includes surrounding yourself with positive individuals who make you laugh out loud or lift your spirits, especially when you are having tough days. You cannot do it alone. This can be in your immediate community or in a virtual community, wherever you receive compassion, understanding, and kindness. Take time to reflect on joyful moments or relationships in your life. This will increase your coping skills during difficult days when you are filled with doubt that you will get better or you are frustrated with joint pain or your daily life. There will be tough days; you know that. Do not hesitate to reach out to someone you trust when you need to share your pain, frustration, or despair.

Embrace other healing arts that are supportive on an emotional and spiritual level. When we wish to heal, it is not only about our physical body. Our emotional body and mind must be part of this complex journey. Past traumatic experiences must be addressed because they play an important role in our ability to become well. Family constellations, shamanic healing, hypnosis, energy healing, homeopathy, and meditation are helpful at this level.

Instead of thinking of yourself as a chronic Lyme patient, reset your thinking. Become proactive in the self-care areas of your life where you *do* have control.

Taking care of your digestive tract and adrenal glands will go a long way; your efforts will be worth it because you will have more energy than before. Give your body a break by decreasing toxic environmental exposures as best as you can. Should you learn just one tip in this book that makes your health change for the better, then writing it was worth it for me. Becoming well is neither a race nor is it linear. In everyone's life, there are always curveballs along the way.

Experiencing small changes for the better on a daily basis are the rainbows we seek, and these provide the motivation to show up every day, on good days and bad days. Take a step back and observe yourself with kindness and love, not judgment and frustration. You are doing your best; take comfort in that.

I invite you to read about the landscape of chronic Lyme in the next chapter. Having a good understanding of the labyrinth of Lyme will make it easier to chart your unique healing strategy. The more you know and the more tools you acquire in your toolbox to handle your own sickness, the more you increase your body's ability to tolerate treatment and to live with the infections—and that is empowering.

"We cannot direct the wind, but we can adjust the sails."

—UNKNOWN

Chapter Two

The Landscape of Persistent Lyme—

A Functional and Holistic Perspective

When it comes to the landscape of chronic Lyme, I always ask my new clients, "Who are you? What was your health like before the infection? Who is currently treating your Lyme or mold-associated illness? What was your life like before you felt ill? Were you born via a natural birth or C-section? Were you breastfed or bottle-fed? Did you often play outside as a child, or did you spend your growing-up years in sanitized homes and school buildings? Do you have your tonsils? How frequently have you used antibiotics (during childhood and in recent years)? Do you exercise or play sports? Do you spend more time indoors or outside? Who is supporting you emotionally during this time (e.g., your partner, family, or friends)? Is there anything that is easing your symptoms right now? Do you eat organic or commercial foods? Does your diet contain animal proteins, or is it plant based? What are your personal goals? How do you feel today? In addition, are there any medications you are taking that might be siphoning away nutrients your body desperately needs? What has been the most traumatic event in your life?" All of these factors are important.

These intake questions provide an important backdrop for the unique individual dealing with persistent Lyme-related symptoms. In conjunction with the above questions, other factors to consider include the medical history of the individual's parents, past and present physical pains, any current injuries, prior digestive troubles, thyroid dysfunction, results of their most recent lab work, childhood vaccinations, emotional traumas, surgeries, psychological troubles, relationship stress, financial worries, seasonal or pet allergies, and chemical sensitivities. All these mind-body layers are important when dealing with the complexities of Lyme-related or environmental illnesses, chronic pain, and auto-immune challenges.

It is not about the illness; it is about the individual, the whole person, whose biography, present biology, genetic potential, immune system, and stressed mind-set are all interwoven with the challenges the illness presents in their daily lives.

Stress of any kind is processed in the body at hormonal, metabolic, and bio-chemical levels. Living in chronic stress mode is very detrimental to our health; sustained stress depletes the body of its nutrient reserves, which are often defi-cient already. A malnourished and tired body will not be able to fight infections.

Hormonal Compensation and Lyme

We are designed to live with short-term stress followed by periods of recovery and rest with the help of the calming parasympathetic nervous system. Being in balance, with acute stress followed by rest, is called *healthy stress adaptation*. But with sustained inflammation from excessive environmental toxins, unhealthy foods, and Lyme-related infections, the body experiences insufficient rest and repair because it remains in fight-or-flight mode. This directly impacts our energy, blood sugar balance, fertility, sleep, and the ability to heal. The body is not concerned with those functions when it is in survival mode. Hormonal imbalances make Lyme symptoms worse, as they are closely connected with our nervous system, digestion, moods, and immune function.

The good news is that our body is always looking out for us; it is continually adapting or compensating to ensure our survival. In its innate wisdom, the body creates resources to fight infections, but it comes with a price. . . . For instance, when it is challenged with chronic infections, the body will resort to using build-ing materials meant for sex hormones, such as progesterone or testosterone, for the production of stress hormones, such as cortisol. However, lower levels of DHEA, testosterone, progesterone, and estrogen, contribute to depression, anxiety, sleep problems, and increased pain and inflammation.

When living with chronic Lyme or mold-related illnesses, the sex and steroid hormones are often out of balance, but there are many treatment options available. Some individuals respond well to hormone replacement therapy; others prefer glandulars, herbals, and homeopathy to support hormonal balance that is closely interlinked with the immune system. I recommend avoiding all synthetic hormones and only choosing a bioidentical option if you opt for hormone replacement therapy.

In those with persistent Lyme, the menstruation cycle is often affected, and even the cessation of menses can occur. With lower sex hormones, the libido is diminished, which can create conflict in personal relationships. Hormonal imbalances with symptoms such as PMS, insomnia, and migraines add other dimensions to an already complex Lyme scenario. Infertility, low sperm counts, or repeated miscarriages are also a concern.

Functional testing from specialized labs is very helpful to gain additional information about the hormonal status in your body. *But it is only as good as its interpretation within the context of clinical findings, and if the appropriate action is taken by your practitioner or doctor.* Testing from specialized labs can be expensive, and the financial aspect can be restrictive and prohibitive for many because these tests are often not covered by insurance companies. Integration of hormonal balance is an important factor when living with the ongoing stress of Lyme disease, yet it is often neglected.

Your Resilience Reservoir = Your Microbiome

Think of your gut flora like an abundant garden full of many different plants (microbes). In a garden, we need healthy soil with diverse strains and species of microorganisms so that we can grow nutrient-dense, healthy plants. With appropriate water, sunlight, and nutrients from the soil, the plants are able to ward off pests, harmful yeasts, and excessive weeds. A healthy soil has its own checks and balances that support nutrient absorption and growth and ward off harmful bugs in the soil.

It is the same with our gut. We need a healthy foundation with a diverse ecology so that the bad microbes do not overrun the good ones. We require a diversity of microbes, yeasts, and bacteria for absorption of nutrients. For every human cell, there are ten microbial cells.

Our gut houses up to seventy percent of our immune system, so we must make sure that we have many more health-supporting microbes than harmful microbes, such as *Candida albicans*. Microbes include over 100 trillion bacteria, parasites, viruses, and fungi, and they form a large part of our microbiota, which is involved in every function of the body.

We used to think in the terms of good bugs and bad bugs, or pathogens; however, this thinking has changed. Now, there is an emphasis on reestablishing the diversity and balance of the internal milieu. Undesired migrations within the digestive tract and overcrowding of any strains of microbes can induce digestive troubles and illness. For example, we harbor strep, staph, and *C. difficile* microbes as normal microbial flora in our colon or *Candida* in our oral cavity.[1] If these are kept in check by a strong immune system and an acidic pH, infections will not have a chance to flourish and the host remains asymptomatic. If the delicate microflora balance becomes disturbed with stress and pH changes, hormonal imbalances, infections, junk foods, or medications, various symptoms and fatigue begin to appear. It is about the terrain.

Microbes in the gut convert the food we eat into vitamins the body can easily use. If we eat foods that were grown in healthy soil, the innate immune microorganisms in the soil and plants come into our body, and they help our immune system. Each section of the gut has its own community of health-supporting microbes, called *commensal microbes*, that perform needed functions.

This is all part of the new information we have learned through the Human Microbiome Project, a five-year project initiative sponsored by the National Institutes of Health. It was launched in 2008, and the goal was to identify microorganisms that are associated with healthy and diseased individuals. From 242 healthy participants in the United States, 500 samples were collected. Microorganisms were studied in the mouth, nasal cavity, skin, vagina, gut, and lungs. It was groundbreaking because it revealed, among many other astounding facts, that our microbes contribute more to our survival and wellness than our own genes.

The diversity of gut microbes, or microbiota, is crucial to the health of our bodies and minds. Out of roughly 35,000 microbe species possible, we each carry a unique combination of roughly 1,000 in our gut. We have area-specific microbiomes in the sinuses, lungs, urinary tract, stomach, intestines, skin, and bowels. They each have specific defense functions depending on their location. (The "hygiene hypothesis" and overuse of antibiotics has been shown to be detrimental to our health with increased immune intolerance, antibiotic resistance, and decreased microbial diversity.[2])

Antibiotics can be lifesaving in that they destroy infectious agents, but they also alter the amount of health-promoting microbes. One round of antibiotic treatment can severely alter the overall microbial balance, allowing harmful yeasts to proliferate. Microbial overgrowth and a lack of diversity in the gut flora cause health problems that can mimic Lyme symptoms.

Whatever we eat, the microbes in our gut eat too. Harmful microbes eat sugar for their energy, and they can induce carb cravings. They are affected by our emotional or psychological stress, and they know when the defense system in the gut is down. Harmful microbes exchange their DNA with other microbes, and they excel at recruiting other microbes when the immune system is weakened. Simply put, they gang up so they can establish dominance by crowding out other strains. After colonization, they proliferate rapidly if they are not reigned in by health-supporting microbes or reduced in numbers with therapeutic treatment. When living with any chronic Lyme-related condition, maintaining flora diversity in the gut is a primary concern, whether you are in therapeutic treatment or not. It is all about checks and balances.

Harmful bacteria, worms, flukes, parasites, protozoa, and amoebas can enter our body through foods we eat, water we drink, and lakes and streams we might swim or wade in. Eating under-cooked or raw foods increases the risk of food-borne infections, especially when there is a lack of hydrochloric acid and lowered immune function in the gut.

Gut microbes in the microbiome are proactive in regulating an overactive immune system and in modulating inflammation. This immune training (hopefully) occurs during the early years with exposure to dirt, childhood illnesses, and playing outside. Formula baby foods, sugary juices, excessive antiseptics, antibiotics, and vaccinations are all known inhibitors of a diverse and tolerant gut microbiology.[3] This microbial programming sets the tone for appropriate immune responses and tolerance of multiple stressors in adolescent and adult life.

If the flora in the gut is diverse, the body can more effectively deal with external infectious agents, while also maintaining a balance of power by crowding out internal microbial overgrowth. The unique gut flora blueprint, or microbiome—

- Is mostly inherited from our mother
- Is established roughly by the age of two
- Plays a very important role in our immune function, resilience, hormonal balance, and food tolerance
- Is greatly affected by foods, medications, and infections
- Is directly connected to our moods and mental wellness
- Is considered our "second brain," due to the presence of neural tissue

It only takes one severe chemical insult, injury, surgery, or emotional stress exposure to tip the balance.

Consideration of your gut flora and gut lining integrity is crucial when it comes to helping you rebound from sickness. Any medications, antibiotics in foods, birth control pills, vaccinations, or emotional shock can severely compromise the commensal gut flora that we require to thrive after a long illness. Eating a clean diet free of refined sugars or processed foods is a fundamental step in aiding our beneficial gut flora and keeping down the population of opportunistic microbes such as *Candida*.

Drainage and Detoxification

How well can your body get rid of toxins? Did you have chemical sensitivities before you were infected with Lyme? Or did you exhibit skin problems, have environmental allergies, or experience headaches in certain situations (e.g., when you were at a gas station)? These symptoms indicate underlying detox weaknesses that are exacerbated by the Lyme infection and mold exposures. The

Lyme infection and toxic exposures could have triggered a cascade of chemical sensitivity because of an already compromised immune system.

An individual's ability to detox is a major factor in how the body handles the burden of Lyme and coinfections and how it responds to therapeutic interventions when dealing with vector-borne infections, viruses, or mold illness. This must be seen in context with the onslaught of factory-produced toxic pollution in our air, food supply, soil, oceans, and rainwater. All of these toxins can accumulate in the body, and, thus, we must be proactive in helping our bodies to get rid of them. If toxins are not eliminated, they build up, which can cause or contribute to Lyme-like symptoms such as palpitations, joint pain, skin eruptions, or headaches. The kidneys and liver are both major elimination channels; however, we must also include the skin, colon, lungs, and lymph as important detoxification pathways. If one channel is clogged, the body will attempt to use other channels. It is not just infections that create health problems; it is also the accumulated chemical toxins from the environment that trigger low-grade and sustained inflammation, which keeps us sick.

With any type of antimicrobial therapeutic treatment, die-off poisons from the microbes are released into the body. These toxins, if not metabolized and eliminated efficiently, create debilitating symptoms, or a herx reaction. Think of it like a clogged pipe under the kitchen or bathroom sink that eventually results in a messy overflow because it does not drain properly. When toxins build up in the body because of lack of drainage, there is a similar reaction. Toxins are reabsorbed and end up in the bloodstream, and the reaction can be so severe that therapeutic treatment must be discontinued. Lymph drainage supporters and binding agents help suck up toxins like a sponge sucks up water. Skin reactions, severe headaches, insomnia, increased pain, nausea, flu-like symptoms, and severe fatigue are common when toxins are not properly eliminated; in severe cases involving anaphylaxis, hospitalization is required. These are symptoms of autointoxication. Whether you're in active treatment or not, it is essential to support the drainage of the lymph fluid between cells where infections and toxins accumulate. *No therapeutic treatment should be implemented without first introducing drainage and detoxification into the protocol.*

Try your best to avoid commercial foods that are sprayed excessively with harmful, cancer-causing pesticides (e.g., herbicides, insecticides, and fungicides). Some foods, such as lettuce and strawberries, are sprayed up to forty-five times before they make their way to your plate. Simply washing produce is not sufficient to remove all the pesticides and chemicals that inflame our body, harm our brain and thyroid, make us gain weight by affecting our insulin levels, and adversely alter our hormones. It is best to eat organic whole foods to lower the toxin exposure in your diet.

Every cell in the body needs clean water to function—not tap water, which contains chlorine, fluoride, lead, arsenic, and other harmful agents. It is best to use filtered water or water that has been purified through reverse osmosis, but do add minerals back in. Water enables communication between the cells, the transport of nutrients into the cells, and the transfer of toxic materials out of the cells. Water-soluble toxins are eliminated through the kidneys, and fat-soluble toxins leave through the stool. With heavy metal detox and chronic infections, especially when taking antibiotics, it is important to consider the role of the kidneys in detox. Teas that are red, such as hibiscus, rooibos, or cranberry, help nourish and support the kidneys.

Any toxin you smell, breathe, or put on your skin will ultimately end up in your liver and brain. Toxins from chemicals, commercial foods, and infections damage cell membranes, irritate the immune system, harm the glands, and adversely affect energy production at the cellular level.

Harmful industrial pollutants are dispersed in the soil, water, and air and cause havoc in our bodies, the oceans, and our wildlife. These harmful chemicals are known as *persistent organic pollutants* and include PCBs, DDT, and dioxins. They are excessive in the environment and have an adverse effect on everyone to some degree. Regulation of these pollutants is greatly insufficient, and profit-driven interests are flourishing at the expense of our physical and mental health. Even babies are born with over two hundred known toxic chemicals in their bloodstream—some of which are known cancer-causing toxins.

Over a lifetime, even a person with healthy liver function is challenged by low-grade, long-term exposure to environmental pollutants, chemicals, plastics, antibiotics, and pesticides. They contribute to cancer (especially in children), autism spectrum-related disorders, autoimmune diseases, infertility, obesity, CIRS (chronic immune response syndrome), mast cell disorders, and neurological illnesses. Our body is not designed to handle the toxic onslaught of the twenty-first century, and, sadly, many more chemical toxins are released into our world everyday.

The toxic burden of cleaning products must be considered, because they too accumulate in the body and brain. Use of commercial household cleaners, detergents, carpet shampoos, and air fresheners add to our internal burden. They disrupt thyroid and reproductive hormones, contributing to biochemical, respiratory, and metabolic disruptions. By making changes to the products you buy, you can decrease your toxic exposures. For home cleaning products, scan the green aisle in your local store or look online and check out the variety of eco-friendly home cleaning products. Our bodies are not designed to handle all these chemicals, especially when liver and gallbladder function are already challenged by chronic infections and medications.

Check your beauty and personal care products and eliminate commercial products that contain harmful chemicals. This is a significant step toward decreasing toxic exposures. Replenish your personal care with organic products that contain at least eighty percent fewer toxins than commercial products. A good resource is the Environmental Working Group website (ewg.org), which rates consumer products. For fragrances to be used on your body or in your home, consider essential oils that calm your stress, lift your energy, and resonate within you. (Note: Most essential oils will need to be diluted with a carrier oil to prevent skin irritation. Even then, a patch test on the inside of your wrist is a good idea.)

Common toxic ingredients in cosmetics, fragrances, and personal-care products include chemical estrogens such as xenoestrogens, benzenes, formaldehyde, aluminum, petroleum, mercury in eye shadows, parabens, bisphenol A, coal tar, phthalates, propylene glycol, sodium lauryl sulfate, talc, synthetic colors and fragrances, and xenobiotics (chemical hormones). Dioxins are found in many commercial cotton balls, tissues, sanitary pads, and tampons, which all come in close contact with our skin and membranes and irritate the immune system. Choose very carefully what you put on your skin; after all, it is the largest detox organ of the body.

When you put these toxins in your hair or on your body, they eventually end up in your bloodstream. If you paint your fingernails, you will inhale toxic vapor. These toxins combine and accumulate into a toxic soup that inflames the body and brain if your body cannot get rid of it.

Becoming aware and limiting your exposure to toxins is a major step in whole body health. If you do not make positive changes in your nutrition, personal care, and home cleaning products, you will continue to poison your body.

Detoxification is often not addressed sufficiently in Lyme treatment; many only think of it in regards to bowel movements. Low-grade accumulation of toxic loads in the lymph fluid that surrounds our cells creates an inflammatory burden. This toxic sludge affects all systems of the body. The good news is that there are various ways you can help your body get rid of toxins.

Herbal Lyme treatment protocols that incorporate detoxification and drainage include the Cowden protocol, Buhner, Beyond Balance, BioBotanical Research products, Energetix, the Byron White protocol, Researched Nutritionals, German Biologics, the Zhang protocol with Chinese herbs, and Dr. Klinghardt's biological treatment of Lyme disease. There are many more, and I urge you to add lymphatic drainage into your daily regime. Acupuncture and Chinese medicine as well as osteopathic, craniosacral, and energetic healing modalities are very helpful in supporting drainage and detoxification. These can include Emotional Freedom Technique, the Rife machine, Reiki, Family Constellations, vibrational healing, and laser therapies. No matter what therapies you choose to treat your unique situation, make sure that appropriate and customized detoxification is part of your program at all times.

You can take an active part in this challenging journey toward optimal detoxification. The more environmental toxins, medications, and dead debris from infections that can be metabolized and eliminated, the better you will feel. It is advisable to do so in small steps, starting with eating predominantly whole foods as tolerated.

On the table that follows, write a checkmark next to each exposure that applies to you. The accumulative effect of all triggers and toxic exposures are important.

Toxic Exposures: The Broad Perspective
Within the Landscape of Chronic Lyme

» Check off your daily exposures

☐ Commercial cleaning products at home

☐ Stick-free pans or plastic cooking utensils

☐ Commercial personal care products, including makeup, deodorant, hair, and skin products

☐ Use of microwave (especially plastic in the microwave)

☐ Commercial dry cleaning

☐ Live in a densely populated, high traffic area such as New York or LA

☐ Water damage at home or work

☐ Need for coffee, sugar, or carbohydrates during the day or at night

☐ Use of artificial sweeteners

☐ Drinking tap water, particularly out of plastic bottles

☐ Consumption of gluten-containing foods

☐ Skip breakfast or other meals during the day

☐ Consumption of nonfat foods or try to avoid fat

☐ Commercially processed foods at work or home (including diet soda, sweet coffee drinks, fried foods, or deli meats)

☐ Smoking

☐ Alcohol use

☐ Lack of exercise

☐ Wi-Fi exposure at home and work, including sitting at computers, and from cell towers and power lines

☐ Stress in personal relationships

☐ Death of a loved one

☐ Bloating, discomfort, indigestion

☐ PMS or symptoms connected with menopause

☐ Lack of sleep or feeling tired during the day

☐ Skin problems

☐ Constipation

☐ Amalgam filling and root canals

☐ Getting an annual flu shot

☐ Use of birth control pills or copper IUD

☐ Excess bodyweight

☐ Removal of gallbladder

☐ Known genetic weaknesses

☐ Skin challenges

☐ Chronic joint pains or cramping

☐ Trouble sleeping

☐ Financial worries

☐ Past abuse (verbal, sexual, emotional, physical, or psychological)

☐ Surgical scars on the body

☐ Use of prescription meds, anti-inflammatories, OTC acid reflux & allergy pills

☐ Recurring yeast infections

☐ Trouble concentrating, feeling anxious and scattered, poor memory

☐ Drink iced drinks or cold water with meals

☐ Vector-borne infections

Biological Dentistry and Metal Toxicity

The mouth is a gateway to the body. Thus, we should make sure that we have a good defense system in place in the mouth. Lyme-related microbes can infest in a root canal or other cavitation. A variety of metals in your mouth from past or current dental work can contribute to symptoms that mimic mold- and Lyme-related illnesses. Dental toxicity can increase neurological symptoms, cognition, and behavioral problems associated with persistent Lyme, *Ehrlichia*, and *Bartonella* infections. You might have symptoms but are not considering a possible infection in the teeth. Dental work that includes the removal of a tooth can expose a hidden Lyme infection, resulting in a serious flare-up. Sinus infections, which may be connected to dental work and root canals, can contribute to ongoing dizziness, vision loss, ear aches, headaches, and balance problems. Every tooth in the mouth is connected to an organ or gland, and the materials used in crowns, braces, and titanium implants can aggravate your immune system and short-circuit your meridians (nerve pathways).

A biological dentist supports your wellness by considering the interconnection between your bite, gum, mouth, nutrition, infections, metal toxicity, and systemic health. Do consider the lymphatic system in the brain is activated by chewing, just like our skeletal muscles activate the lymphatic system when we exercise. The muscles of the jaw and face interact with the brain during chewing. With chronic Lyme or mold infection, or any neurological symptoms, we have to drain an inflamed and toxic brain. During the day, massage your face, neck, and throat muscles with arnica and engage in oil pulling with coconut oil to stimulate detox and drainage activity. (Consider using a splint at night when you sleep to support drainage and breathing.) Your bite, teeth, and mouth can contribute to hidden immune and mental challenges. Biological dentists can also decrease your risk of exposures to toxic dental materials and X-rays that can contribute to, or mimic, Lyme-related symptoms.

The mouth is filled with health-supporting microbes that create a naturally occurring slimy layer coating our teeth and gums. This is known as *biofilm*, and it is part of our oral microbiome. Immune cells in our saliva fight harmful pathogens that come in through the foods we eat, the air we breathe, and the secretions that drip down from our noses. Refined sugars, processed foods, and harmful chemical substances (including fluoride in drinking water or toothpaste or commercial oral antiseptic mouthwashes with artificial colors and chemicals) all harm our oral flora because they destroy the health-supporting microbes in our mouths. Look after these helpful microbes; after all, they are looking after you.

Removal of silver amalgam fillings must be done by a biological dentist, one who uses a special technique that reduces leaking of toxic mercury vapors into the brain when removing the fillings. Mercury is of great concern, especially with amalgam fillings that leach vapors into the brain and heart. Before amalgam removal, consult with a biological dentist and the doctor who is treating you for Lyme to discuss the timing and spacing of these procedures. This matters greatly and certain drainage supplements and binders must be part of the amalgam removal protocol.

Heavy metal and metal toxicity from fillings, crowns, braces, and root canals can also cause health problems. The metals have an electric charge just like the brain, heart, and nervous system. Any misfiring or short-circuiting when metals touch each other (e.g., gold and mercury under a porcelain crown) can dysregulate the entire nervous system. This affects the function of every gland and organ, especially the heart. It is helpful to seek out a holistic dentist who understands the impact of metals in the mouth, disruption of the oral flora, root canals, and titanium implants in their relationship to environmental illness and your symptoms.

Should braces be needed, it is best to first consult with an osteopath who also assesses the overall posture, the skull, the bite, and other important face, head, and neck structures. As an alternative to commercial braces, which can be toxic, consider Advanced Lightwire Functionals (ALF). It is best to work with an orthodontist who understands the implications of crowded teeth in children and the dangers of metals in the mouth and body.

Root canals can aggravate Lyme-related infections because they become sites for other infections, called *foci infections*. The immune system cannot maintain surveillance, and the root canal is a great hiding place for these infections, which increase low-grade inflammation and the risk of neurological symptoms, strokes, and cardiovascular disease. If you are making significant therapeutic and wellness changes but your Lyme-related symptoms aren't improving, it's possible that amalgam fillings, root canals, crowns, retainers, and titanium implants are blocking your health-building journey.

Regularly rinse the mouth with sea salt or consider oil pulling with coconut oil. Make sure to spit out the oil in the trash can and not in the sink because it can clog your pipes. Or use a water pick to support your oral wellness. If you are suffering from a yeast infection in the mouth, you could make an oral probiotic with *Saccharomyces boulardii*, a probiotic, or use an herbal antifungal rinse. Grapefruit seed extract or essential oils diluted in water and used as a rinse can be helpful, or you can use concentrated pau d'arco, which is held in the mouth for a prolonged period. These home therapies are natural antimicrobial and antiseptic modalities.

Use a soft toothbrush and choose fluoride-free toothpaste, unless you make your own with baking soda and essential oils. Use cloves, chlorophyll, oregano oil, or colloidal silver as an antiseptic when you are troubled with an infected tooth or are having dental work done. Your oral health plays an important role in your overall wellness in many ways. Remember that harmful microbes hide below the gum line, so make sure your gums are in good shape, and be aware that flossing can create problems in the gum line.

The Mold Factor

If you live or work in a moldy home or office, frequent a moldy structure (e.g., an old bookstore, church, or library), each time you breathe, you inhale mold spores. These spores also make their way onto your clothes and your belongings, allowing for contamination wherever you go. These mold spores can cause illness, with symptoms similar to those caused by Lyme infections. Many people do not know that these mold spores are what's keeping them ill. They often assume that it's just the Lyme infection.

It is important to understand that mold is only part of the problem. Mold toxins, heavy metal toxicity, genetic factors, underlying respiratory ailments, antibiotic use, a weakened immune system, increased chemical sensitivities, hormonal imbalances, and viral infections are all interconnected. If your immune system is weakened by the Lyme infections and antibiotics (and nonoptimal eating habits), you are more susceptible to fungal overgrowth in the body. You will also be more affected by mold in your environment. Symptoms can mimic Lyme, and Lyme can mimic mold illness.

Many people do not understand how difficult daily life can be for the individual dealing with a toxic mold infection. Misdiagnosed individuals are prescribed multiple prescription drugs, including antidepressants, antipsychotics, and sleep medications—even though they have toxic mold illness. Often, mold-toxic individuals are diagnosed with the vague diagnosis of chronic fatigue syndrome because they are not able to function in daily life.

Indoors, mold is prevalent under older carpets, in sheetrock, in walls, in shower stalls, in basements, and in air conditioner ducts. Water damage in older apartments and homes that was not correctly remediated increases the risk of harmful mold exposures for the people living there. Newer buildings that are energy efficient and not well ventilated can trap toxic mold spores that are inhaled by occupants. Finished and unfinished basements in homes without adequate humidifiers are breeding grounds for mold that can spread quickly through the house during humid and warm months.

Mold spores also exist outdoors. They can be found in the air, soil, and everywhere in nature where it is warm, damp, and humid, including compost piles and wooded areas that favor the growth of mold and mushrooms.

The low-grade but chronic exposure to home and environmental mold causes Lyme and fungus-related symptoms to worsen, especially if you are living in a humid climate with outdoor mold exposures as well. Symptoms include a hyper-reactive immune response, chronic sinusitis, and a metallic taste in the mouth. With mold illness, colonization of multiple antibiotic-resistant microbes, called *macrons* (multiple antibiotic resistant coagulase negative staph colonization), can often occur, and these must be treated before any therapeutic Lyme treatment can begin. Individuals suffering from this condition have no tolerance for exercise. It takes an investigative and integrated approach to address the various components of this complicated and misunderstood environmental illness.

Mold toxins wreak havoc on the brain and the body's biochemistry. The blood-brain barrier is designed to keep toxins out of the sensitive brain; when it is breached, poisonous substances enter the brain and cause damage. This damage causes psychiatric symptoms and learning disabilities that are often misdiagnosed by psychiatrists and pediatricians. For instance, toxic mold illnesses can be misdiagnosed as autism spectrum–related disorders because the symptoms are similar. This is all part of the complex landscape of chronic Lyme.

When suffering from toxic mold exposure, melatonin production is compromised; thus, insomnia is a common occurrence. Sleep patterns are often disrupted, contributing to excessive fatigue as well as neurological, behavioral, and bipolar disorders that are often treated with hard-core drugs from a psychiatric professional without a thorough medical and living-environment evaluation.

Mold toxins also alter the brain, especially the forebrain. Symptoms of a toxic brain can include debilitating brain fog, thinking glitches, headaches, memory and vision problems, severe trigeminal nerve-related migraines, cognitive issues, and obsessive-compulsive behavior. Imagine it like a virus entering your computer—it doesn't work anymore, and the screen is scrambled. This is what happens with mold exposures in the brain. It can be debilitating, causing anxiety, depression, and even the risk of suicide.

If you are not sure if you are suffering from toxic mold exposure, you can do a self-test by leaving your home and moving into a sterile environment, with new clothes, for four to five days. Then, go back home and see how you feel. As long as you are exposed to harmful mold toxins in your home, you are constantly repoisoning your system. As a temporary measure, physicians prescribe BEG spray and cholestyramine to detox mold toxins, but there are other options, such as Argentyn23 and bentonite clay or chlorella; however, to become well, you must get into a mold-free environment. If you choose to move, it is necessary to leave all furniture behind and to have your clothes professionally cleaned to avoid a transfer of spores.

There is no one simple test to know if you have a mold illness. The work of Dr. Richie Shoemaker is instrumental, and his comprehensive book, *Surviving Mold,* is a good resource that discusses the visual aids test, MSH testing, nasal swabs for MARCoNS, inflammatory and genetic blood markers implicated with mold sickness, available mold testing in homes, and remediation techniques.

It is best to use professional remediation to address any mold contamination in the home. Increased exposure to spores and toxic chemicals is a risk, especially without proper precautions. It is worth the money to get it done professionally. Common remediation options include extremely toxic chemicals, but I recommend the biological approach with enzymes.

From a nutritional perspective, food choices beyond dairy and gluten can add fuel to the flame for those with mold illness. Each case is unique and must be treated differently. Refined sugars, processed foods, high-sugar fruits, vegetables, and nuts can feed the fungal infection. Foods and supplements that contain yeast can make mold and Lyme symptoms worse; however, this is currently under debate.

When discussing mold illness, it is important to consider the impact of histamine, which occurs naturally in our bodies and in foods. Chronic infections, medications, and genetic weaknesses can create or contribute to a scenario where the body has difficulty breaking down excess histamine. If this happens, the histamine accumulates in the bloodstream. An excess of histamine-producing gut microbes can also create symptoms that mimic Lyme or mold illness, so the gut flora plays a role as well. (Mast cell disorders are complex and part of a new frontier.) Foods high in histamine (and dairy) are best avoided when mold illness is present.

Prepare foods in smaller batches so that you eat a variety of fresh foods daily and decrease excess food-related histamine exposures. It is best not to leave food out on the counter for too long. Once cooled, store foods (e.g., broth, pureed vegetables, or stews) in glass containers in the freezer. Daily food preparation is a lot of work, so freezing cooked foods can be very helpful, especially since chronic fatigue is a big challenge with mold- or Lyme-related illnesses, and some days you are too tired to prepare a meal from scratch. Go organic, go fresh.

The Chronic Pain Factor

Hidden stealth infections are often the root cause of ongoing pain and sustained inflammation. These factors can contribute to increased blood viscosity and increased risk of strokes and cardiovascular events.[4] Infections include latent viral infections and vector-borne infections, which mimic our own cells in a process called *molecular mimicry*. They play hide-and-go-seek in our joints, organs, and glands, creating sustained inflammation and a prolonged and dysregulated overreaction from the immune system, which becomes more aggressive in going after perceived offenders—even if that includes the cells of our own bodies. When the immune system overreacts and cannot clearly discern between self and nonself, autoimmune diseases can occur.

Many with vector-borne infections are misdiagnosed, and often these individuals are prescribed long-term use of immunosuppressant and chemotherapeutic medications by their rheumatologist, gastroenterologists, or pain management doctors. These will make Lyme-related and chronic fatigue symptoms worse and increase the potential risk of additional illnesses for an already compromised body. Immunosuppressing drugs increase the risk of serious infectious complications, cancer, and liver damage. Roughly ten percent of individuals have continued joint pain after standard antibiotic treatment for Lyme. However, that number is most likely higher because many with prolonged arthritic joint pain and swelling go undiagnosed.[5] A *B. burgdorferi* infection is not even considered a possibility in many cases, especially if initial blood tests are negative. Symptoms can mimic those of osteoarthritis, juvenile arthritis, and rheumatoid arthritis, and pain can manifest in the knees, hips, wrists, elbows, shoulders, and fingers. It is debilitating, and the pain greatly affects quality of life.

Do consider the structural angle in your pain management. The structures of the body are interconnected with your nervous system; thus, misalignment in the bite, neck, and spinal column will worsen your pain symptoms. Your spine works closely with all organs, glands, and the entire nervous system. Chiropractic care, cranial osteopathy, and craniosacral therapy are very valuable when you have experienced physical trauma or had to use braces during childhood. Even our birthing process can alter our structural alignment. I recommend seeking a professional to help you maintain an optimal structural alignment.

Any physical brain injury, including a concussion or whiplash can contribute to pain many years after the injury occurred. An injury can include, for example, a blow to the head or a car accident. Physical head trauma can also contribute to a leaky gut (this is referred to as *intestinal permeability*), making it easier for toxins and infectious microbes to get into the brain.

When Lyme-related infections settle in parts of the brain or on the microglial cells of the vagus nerve that runs along your torso, an inflamed and irritated nervous system can cause increased nerve pain as well as neuralgia and palsy symptoms in the head, face, and digestive tract.

Gut health also plays an important role in helping to alleviate chronic pain. The gut is closely connected to the brain via the vagus nerve. Mysterious muscle pains, such as fibromyalgia pain, are common symptoms with Lyme-associated and viral illnesses, and digestive challenges including small intestinal bacterial overgrowth (SIBO). Hypersensitive nerve cells and inflammation drive the pain cycle in connective tissues. An inflamed gut, elevated oxalate levels, and food intolerances increase joint pain, so consider your daily nutrition and gut health within your pain management strategy.

A challenged hypothyroid and adrenal status will also increase painful symptoms. I recommend getting both appropriately checked by a functional medicine doctor. A lack of essential fatty acids, electrolytes, and dehydration can cause pain as well.

Chemical solvents, electromagnetic exposures, and dietary factors contribute to the worsening of seizures, palsy, nervous ticks, headaches, migraines, trigeminal neuralgia, chemical sensitivities, and more. Vaccinations and flu shots containing harmful chemicals such as formaldehyde, thimerosol, and aluminum and excessive environmental toxins in the soil, food, water, and air all play a role in the current rise in autoimmune diseases, low-grade inflammation, and chronic pain symptoms. Metal toxicity, such as aluminum, which is a common additive in commercial baked goods, baking powders, underarm deodorants, and in atmospheric spraying of chemtrails, is also a factor. Lead in drinking water, as was exposed during the Flint water crisis, and arsenic in white rice contribute to increased inflammation and immune system dysregulation. Smoking, refined sugars, and alcohol use increase toxicity and inflame blood vessels in the body.

These environmental and dietary toxic exposures can alter genes and affect important mechanisms in the body, especially in regards to detoxification pathways, allergies, cardiovascular inflammation, cellular energy production, and brain chemicals. When living with Lyme, any additional chemical or Wi-Fi insult can initiate psychiatric and neurological pain symptoms, activate a dormant retrovirus, or create a flare of joint pain symptoms.[6]

Long-term use of pharmaceutical pain management has consequences. Every pharmaceutical has side effects. I am not against Western Medicine when it comes to acute care, emergency care, or relief care, but it is important to find the least amount of pharmaceutical interventions necessary when managing chronic pain. Commercial medicine and profit-driven interest groups heavily promote vaccinations, powerful and addictive opioids, analgesics, and annual flu shots.

From a nutritional perspective, it is worthwhile to consider the impact of daily nutrition on prolonged pain. Many foods that we consume on a regular basis are pain triggers, especially commercial foods. Foods such as avocado, beets, blueberries, celery, leafy greens, coconut oil, and wild salmon calm the central nervous system, where our pain perception begins. Elimination or restriction of the following foods is essential when suffering from Lyme-arthritic pain:

- Gluten-containing foods include wheat, barley, rye, and spelt. (Oats can be problematic because of cross-contamination as they are often processed with the same equipment used for wheat processing.)
- Dairy-containing foods must also be considered as inflammatory triggers for many individuals, especially with cognition, behavior, mood, and attention disorders.
- Corn can contribute to brain seizures and palsy. Beware of corn oil hidden in processed foods and GMO corn-fed commercially processed animal products, including eggs.
- Be mindful of MSG, high sodium levels, and trans fats in processed foods. All inflame the brain.
- High histamine foods can exacerbate neurological and behavioral symptoms.
- Aspartame and sugar substitutes can cause migraines and seizures. Examples include Equal and NutraSweet, which are prevalent in diet sodas and sugar-free dessert products.
- Soy sensitivity is common. It is often hidden in foods such as soybean oil, soybean lecithin in chocolate, and supplements. Commercially processed soy is a GMO food and is a popular milk substitute and baby formula. Avoid it. Only fermented sources such as natto, tempeh, and miso are acceptable for some individuals.

Lowering inflammation will contribute to improved cognition and focus, stable moods, and better function in daily activities. Herbal therapies, choline, vitamins, amino acids, acetylcarnitine, essential fatty acids, and mineral support (e.g., magnesium theonate, skullcap, L-theanine, and phosphatidylserine) are very helpful in calming the brain and relieving pain. The B vitamins—especially B1, B2, activated B6, various forms of folate, and B12—and minerals play an important role when it comes to pain relief—and improved memory.

The brain relies on microcirculation to deliver nutrients to the inflamed brain. Garlic, ginko, berries, and cod liver oil increase microcirculation and will also benefit the eyes, heart, and kidneys.

Supporting drainage with homeopathic or herbal products decreases pain. Red root, cleavers, burdock, essaic tea, and nettles are available in formulations from various companies. Poke root is powerful but must only be taken with supervision and combined with anti-inflammatories. These include resveratrol, water hyssop, turmeric, ginger, cinnamon, choline, green tea extract, and vinpocetine. Arnica, celery seed, ashwagandha, frankincense, topical magnesium oil, or dimethyl sulfoxide cream are helpful pain relief for joints and muscles. Essential oils including lavender, lemon balm, and chamomile are also helpful, especially if applied at the bottom of the feet at bedtime.

What about cannabis and pain modification? The endocannabinoid system, located in the brain and the central and peripheral nervous systems, impacts every biological and physiological system in the body, including our own internal pain modulation and brain protection. If there is insufficient production of naturally produced endocannabinoids within the body, cannabis oil supplementation can be very helpful for pain management and lowering inflammation naturally.

Cannabis and hemp are regulated differently by the FDA; cannabis is considered a drug, and hemp oil is considered a dietary supplement. Cannabis is classified as a schedule 1 drug by the Drug Enforcement Administration, and this has hampered research and its medicinal availability. Cannabidiol (CBD) in the medical marijuana plant or industrially grown hemp plant does not elicit the psychotropic effect that is sought out by recreational users. In medicinal use of cannabis, CBD and THC can be adjusted according to the benefit an individual seeks and can help with pain relief, alleviating anxiety and nausea, improving sleep, and lifting depressed moods.

Legal status regarding medicinal use of CBD varies from state to state, and it remains illegal in many parts of the world. However, there is currently an FDA-approved clinical trial regarding a pharmaceutical version of CBD for children with epilepsy. This is an exciting field, because CBD has been helpful for many symptoms in many different illnesses. It has shown anti-inflammatory, antipsychotic, antitumor, anticonvulsant, and antioxidant properties in animal studies. Cannabidiol oil with an anti-inflammatory high CBD content has been helpful with neurological pain symptoms and is being studied in neurodegenerative diseases.

Low-dose naltrexone (LDN) is also of great interest when sustained pain, gut issues, and mood symptoms are present. For many, it has been helpful in pain reduction, immune system modulation, lowering of inflammation in the nervous system, and improving mood, sleep, and gut function. LDN was found to have immune-supporting properties in HIV,[7] and clinical results showed it was effective for many in preventing disease progression in multiple sclerosis,[8] though some individuals do not tolerate it. LDN is not covered by insurance. Everyone experiences side effects initially, and the dosage must be fine-tuned. There is currently no data on long-term safety, and research is ongoing for off-label applications.

Various pain treatment options include topical magnesium oils and sprays, arnica, tinctures, epsom salts, castor oil packs, and magnesium foot baths, and they are helpful for cramping, spasms, and pain relief. Essential oils diluted in jojoba or coconut oil provide relief when applied to the bottom of feet at night. Topical dimethyl sulfoxide (DMSO) has been shown to provide effective relief for Lyme arthritic-type joint pain as it reduces inflammation by several mechanisms. It can take a few weeks before the effect is felt. (I have seen good results on my scars in just a few days.) Stress-reduction techniques that help calm the brain include deep breathing, meditation, biofeedback modalities, grounding, listening to classical music, watching the flame from a candle, and laughter. Everyone is different, so choose what resonates with you, but make sure you include laughter in your day.

The Genetic Factor

We inherit our unique genes from our mom and dad. Some are good and some are not so good; we hope those that are not so good stay dormant. The body learns to compensate if certain genetic mechanisms are not working well. Nutrition, lifestyle, and good gut flora diversity can keep inherited harmful genes silent. However, environmental toxins, stress, electromagnetic exposures, vaccinations, mold exposures, junk foods, and any infections can turn them on; then symptoms of ill health will appear, including cancers, diabetes, and mood disorders. This phenomenon is called *epigenetics*. This is where the focus must be placed—not on the genes. Genetics are just one player in the ballgame, and challenges must be addressed with targeted nutrients to support genetic detox weaknesses.

With Lyme, inherited genetic vulnerabilities, or glitches, often come into play, and they can affect the immune system's ability to fight off infections. Think of these genetic vulnerabilities as weak links. A Lyme infection, traumatic event, surgery, or chronic, toxic mold exposure can change the ballgame. When switched on, they create a problem in how well cells function at the biochemical and metabolic levels. In addition, an important biochemical process called *methylation* does not work well. This can severely compromise one's ability to get rid of toxins, while increasing the risk of food sensitivities, allergies, mood disorders, and various degenerative diseases.

Methylation is a process in which the body neutralizes and gets rid of toxins. It occurs in all the cells, but primarily in the liver. Think of the liver as a large warehouse where toxins are stored before being processed. In the biochemical process called methylation, there are two phases.

In the first phase chemical toxins, xenobiotics, and heavy metals are broken down into smaller molecules, which are now extremely toxic; they are called *free radicals*. This is known as the cytochrome P450 pathway, and it is adversely affected by many medications. This complex pathway involves many enzymes that function like construction workers; they make things happen. Pesticides, medications, alcohol, exhaust fumes, and so on all create challenges that can inhibit important enzyme functions. Also, bacterial infections in the gut release toxins called *lipopolysaccharides* (LPS), which interfere with this phase of liver detox. Now chemical pollutants, estrogens, and pesticides can accumulate in the body. Some individuals have genetic weaknesses in this initial pathway, making it more difficult for the body to metabolize and eliminate toxins. It is not just about Lyme.

During phase two, super-toxic substances are converted into a less-toxic form. This repackaging of toxins occurs in the presence of enzymes, vitamins, and minerals. Various complex processes occur until the now less-toxic molecules are "wrapped up" and released into the bile. This is one reason why it is necessary to pay attention to gallbladder function, as it plays an important role in the body's ability to get rid of toxins.

Water-soluble toxins will be eliminated through the kidneys, and fat-soluble toxins will be eliminated through the colon. Toxins are also eliminated through the skin (sweat) and lungs (gasses or mucous). These are our organs of elimination. If there is a blockage in one, the body will choose another, and this might lead to a skin outbreak or respiratory ailment, for example.

Genetic testing can shed light on your ability to get rid of toxins and chemical estrogens, which can cause other problems beyond the Lyme infection. Some genetic tests are covered by insurance and some are not. Specialized genetic tests can indicate, not diagnose, possible genetic vulnerabilities, such as the 23andMe test. Commercial foods, stress, PTSD, toxins, and infections can be epigenetic triggers. Your medical history and clinical test results can provide adjunct information regarding genetic implications. If genetic weaknesses are found, targeted supplementation is recommended to improve function. Genetic vulnerabilities can make it more difficult—even up to seventy percent—for the body to process and eliminate toxins. And with vector-borne infections and biotoxin illness from mold exposures, this greatly impacts an individual's ability to become well. The toxic and inflammatory burden causes biochemical havoc; it is not just the Lyme infection.[9]

If the fuel from our daily nutrition is deficient, the body will not have the nutrients it needs for biochemical processes involved in detox. Eating a whole-food diet rich in plants, animal foods, and some fruits is vital; a deficiency of vitamin C, vitamin E, vitamin B6, selenium, zinc, magnesium, B12, folate, glutathione, molybdenum, and trace minerals will impede your ability to get rid of toxins.

Our nutrient intake from the foods we eat is often not enough for the body to function properly. Also, the stress from chronic Lyme (and medications) depletes many of the body's nutrient reserves, which might already be at suboptimal levels. As a result, toxic waste and heavy metals accumulate, and organs and glands function at a subpar level. We feel exhausted, sick, and overwhelmed; we gain weight and cannot think clearly.

If you are under medical care, connect with your Lyme physician and discuss testing for pyrrole disorder, which affects zinc, vitamin B6, manganese, and magnesium in particular. This must be considered before beginning any therapeutic treatment for vector-borne infections. A deficiency in these nutrients, which can be genetically based or acquired because of chronic infections, can have severe neurological and behavioral effects besides impeding any chance of becoming better after ongoing illness. Higher therapeutic doses and activated nutrients are required (e.g., high dosages of vitamin B6 in a more bioavailable ready-to-use form, such as pyridoxal phosphate and zinc, but beware of possible copper imbalances). There are tests for pyrrole disorder available online; however, treatment of this condition must *only* be done with professional supervision because high-dose supplementation must be titrated according to how the individual responds.

Let's Talk About Lifestyle

Our lifestyle plays an important role in our energy, immune function, and mood. We must take care of ourselves every day. If you overdo it, get upset, or get too stressed out, you feel wiped out. You have unique needs to consider when navigating through your individual daily landscape.

NONFATIGUE-INDUCING EXERCISE AND POST-EXERCISE REST

The symptoms from Lyme-associated infections are different for each individual. Some experience painful joints, and others do not. Some experience seizures and terrible insomnia; others do not. Just as personalized medicine and personalized nutrition are key to your wellness, so it is with exercise. Taking fatigue, heat sensitivity, and individual Lyme-associated symptoms into consideration, it is essential to support strength training and flexibility for daily activities. Incorporating a modified exercise program with gentle or moderate movement, as tolerated, will improve function, lymphatic flow, and moods, while also decreasing pain. (With mold-related illness, exercise will make symptoms worse, and aerobic exercise is contraindicated.)

After exercising, apply magnesium oil or arnica oil to tight and cramping muscles. For chronic joint pain and stiff muscles, a warm shower before exercise can be beneficial as well. Improved circulation with nonfatigue-inducing exercise can make the muscles more pliable, and this will bring more ease to daily activities. With gentle movements, you will hopefully feel the tension leave your body and mind as you are present with your breath.

It is best to avoid any prolonged activity that elevates the heart rate and raises the body temperature so you feel uncomfortable and symptomatic. Avoid exercising at the time of day when you feel the most tired. With Lyme, it is important to schedule a period of rest after completion of exercise or physical therapy.

With weight training, include a higher number of repetitions with low resistance in each set. Oxygen and blood flow will increase in the area with repetitive motions. This will decrease arthritis-type pains, increase healing metabolic activity in the cells, and facilitate removal of toxins in the lymphatic tissues. And you will feel better too. The repetitive movement with a gentle pumping action releases tight or tense muscles, increasing desired range of motion at the joints. Be sure to rest afterwards.

Full-body exercises support function in daily activities, including carrying a shopping bag, getting in and out of a car, or emptying the dishwasher. Because they require energy, posture, and balance, standing exercises are more demanding than seated machine or mat work on the floor, so take your fatigue, balance, and pain into consideration with these types of exercises. To avoid fatigue, it is best to begin with a few isolation exercises that use single muscles and joints. From there, gradually build in more exercises but do not push too hard. Listen to your body and only do what you can tolerate that day.

When persistent Lyme infections affect balance, vision, and the inner ear, exercises in a controlled environment, where the risk of falling is minimized, are helpful. To reduce risks but still support the building of muscle, using weight machines and doing exercises while seated are recommended. Low-grade cardiovascular conditioning can be achieved on a stationary bike or in the pool, if walking is not an option. However, *fatigue must always be considered* because exercise is stress on the body; it can push the body into fight-or-flight mode if the program is too intense. Neurological training with exercises on the floor, such as Feldenkrais, or careful use of the Swiss ball or foam roller are helpful to communicate with an errant nervous system in addressing reflex mechanisms at joint level. Muscle atrophy, bone loss, and lack of overall strength is of concern, especially with digestive troubles, malnourishment, and decreased sex hormones.

If weight loss is desired, appropriate weight training and walking short intervals throughout the day supports insulin sensitivity and metabolic function. Weight training uses up sugar (glycogen) in the muscles, and it induces a hormonal and brain chemical response that can provide more energy, pain reduction, and mental clarity.

Exercise also improves mitochondrial function (the energy center of cells), and it actually helps increase the number of mitochondria in the exercising muscles. Increased mitochondrial function supports all functions in the body.

With heat intolerance that can occur with some Lyme-related infections, movement modalities in a cool place, such as gentle stretching, Pilates, or hatha yoga done at home in a controlled environment, might be more appropriate.

If any fluoroquinolone antibiotics such as ciprofloxacin or levofloxacin are in play, be very careful. Tendon ruptures are common when taking these medications. This type of antibiotic also affects the central nervous system and can induce insomnia, headaches, dizziness, anxiety, hallucinations, and acute psychosis.[10] *Often, patients are not advised of these side effects when these antibiotics are prescribed.*

The Power of Sleep and Rest

It sounds strange, but you must be able to sleep to get a good night's rest. Living in stress mode and fighting infections interrupts the natural day and night waking and sleeping pattern called the *circadian rhythm*. In this cycle, the daytime hormone (cortisol) and the nighttime hormone (melatonin) alternate within a twenty-four-hour cycle that is primed to make us highly functional during the day, with repair and organ restoration during sleep at night.

Maybe you have trouble falling asleep quickly; perhaps you have night fevers or sweats, have heart palpitations, feel wired and stay up past midnight, are in pain, worry about how you will get through this, or have a restless night—all will leave you tired in the morning. Many people cannot fall asleep and feel more awake at night. Over time, this results in hormonal disruptions that can have debilitating consequences.

With chronic Lyme and other infections, sleep is often compromised, yet sleep is one of the body's most powerful tools for supporting our immune system. Infections also interfere with brain chemicals and hormones, including melatonin (our sleeping hormone) and cortisol. Lack of sleep keeps the body agitated in the sympathetic nervous system's fight-or-flight response, and increased fatigue and inflammation, weight gain, mood disorders, and blood sugar and insulin imbalances are often a result.

It is during sleep that our brain does its housekeeping and rids itself of toxins. The brain cells shrink. During sleep, the lymphatic system can flow freely in the extracellular spaces and toxins can be cleared from the brain. This is also known as the *glymphatic system* because it involves the waste-clearing action of glial cells and the lymphatic system in the brain.[11] This occurs during different cycles in our sleep. If sleep is interrupted or too short, this vital "brain drain" function cannot occur. This causes toxic build-up in the brain, which is implicated in many illnesses and mood and behavior disorders, including autism and degenerative diseases.[12]

Adrenal function becomes challenged as the body and mind are under constant stress. Worrying if you will get palpitations or if you're getting worse only drives fear. The adrenal glands become drained just like a car battery, resulting in decreased output of cortisol.

With the constant strain from Lyme-related infections, the amount of cortisol secreted from the adrenal glands is often insufficient to assist in steady blood sugar regulation during the night. This might be the reason why you wake with hypoglycemia (low blood sugar), even though you ate a good dinner earlier in the evening. Having a snack that consists of protein and carbohydrates before bedtime might be helpful to offset a blood sugar dip during the night; you might also consider something to aid in adrenal support, such as licorice (unless you have elevated blood pressure) or herbal adaptogens, such as ashwagandha or eleuthero.

During sleep, the immune system becomes more active and goes on the hunt for harmful agents. This is one of the reasons why night fevers occur. Infectious microbes (e.g., bacteria, viruses, protozoa, and parasites) become more active during the night—and certain parasites are especially active during the full moon—keeping you up. Nutritional, herbal, and mineral interventions can help; in many cases, a cocktail must be created to facilitate deep, restorative sleep.

The sleeping environment matters, too. It is best to remove all electronics and Wi-Fi from your bedroom, because they impede your sleep. According to scientists, prolonged electromagnetic frequency exposures from mobile and cordless phones, computers, and other electronic devices have adverse health effects. This includes lowered immune function, altered hormonal balance, metabolic and reproductive disturbances, headaches, low melatonin production, slowed reaction times, sleep problems, and changes in brain activity. Electromagnetic frequencies contribute to a leaky brain, and they are a risk factor in Alzheimer's disease. (Pregnant women, babies, and children are especially vulnerable.)[13] They also irritate infectious microbes in vector-borne illnesses, which then become more aggressive. It is best to limit time with the computer or other electronic devices and to keep electronic devices away from your head and heart. Both are major centers of electrical activities. Take note of any cell towers in your area and power lines near your residence; these too can make your symptoms worse. Also make sure any smart meters attached to your house are not near your bedroom. Keep the electronic devices away from direct contact with the brain and body. Ideally, keep a landline for phone use at home if possible.

Choose bedding that is organic cotton, and only use green detergent; artificially scented products irritate the body. It takes a multipronged strategy involving stress reduction techniques, dietary measures, supplement cocktails, and addressing the sleep environment when solving chronic Lyme sleep problems.

Sleep medications come with side effects and addiction concerns, and they can make certain symptoms worse in the long run because they do not address root causes. Herbal support can include passionflower, lemon balm, hops, and valerian, but you should discuss their use with a health-care professional. Melatonin, cannabis, or amino acid supplementation, such as 5-HTP or glycine, is helpful for some but not others. Everyone is unique and will respond differently to treatments (genetics come into play here). It is important to find out what works best for you.

With sleep challenges it is important to create rest periods during the day, because you are running on low energy already. See how you can simplify your schedule or commitments to reduce mental and physical stress. Any excess energy expenditure or emotionally stressful event can leave you feeling wiped out, and your symptoms will flare up even worse. Plan your day so you can have daily rest, even if it is only for ten or fifteen minutes. You need it.

Regular stress-reduction techniques will help your ability to sleep. They rebalance the nervous system, moving us from the adrenaline-charged survival brain into the restorative configuration of the parasympathetic nervous system— the calm part of the brain that allows us to sleep, rest, digest, detox, and repair.

Examples include meditation and breathing exercises that can be done at home daily. If you do not know how to begin, perhaps stream an online video guide or purchase a guided meditation that resonates with you. Other modalities support calming the brain, such as HeartMath (a biofeedback technique), and use of essential oils or homeopathic remedies. These stress-reduction techniques are effective as energy-building and detoxification strategies.

Look into your community wellness groups or check out health clubs and yoga studios. Some offer gentle rejuvenation or meditation classes that might give you a needed jump start. They also include social support that you might find helpful to lower your stress and improve your outlook on life. You do not have to do it alone, and you can always consult with a professional who understands the complexity of what you are going through.

. . . .

Wrapping Up

Create your wellness team with professionals from the medical and holistic arenas who you trust to assist you in dealing with the landscape of chronic Lyme. They should communicate with each other regarding your specific needs and obstacles along the way. You can only get well if you trust in your team, your treatment, and your ability to get better.

From a holistic viewpoint, it is important to see the person as a whole, to respect spiritual beliefs, and to support the individual from a mind-body perspective. With all the complexities involved, it is prudent to choose practitioners who have a thorough understanding of the effects of the disease, side effects of treatments, functional physiology, and customized nutrition.

Managing the infections and becoming well takes an integrated team effort; it is a long-term, ongoing process. I am grateful to be involved in my clients' wellness journeys. Having family, professional, and social support is imperative, especially when one is going through very rough times.

"Give yourself a gift of five minutes of contemplation in awe of everything you see around you. Go outside and turn your attention to the many miracles around you. This five-minute-a-day regimen of appreciation and gratitude will help you to focus your life in awe."

—WAYNE DYER

Chapter Three

Eat For Energy

We eat every day, multiple times a day. Through our food choices, we can heal or inflame our body. Often, a healthy eating plan is something we have to relearn, perhaps even learn. It depends on what dietary path we were on growing up.

Did you grow up eating home-cooked meals regularly, or did you eat sugar-filled cereals for breakfast and microwaved dinners on a TV tray? Did you follow a nonfat or low-fat regimen and use artificial sweeteners in an attempt to lose weight? Habits and learned eating behaviors from childhood tend to carry over into our adult lives. We live in a world of dietary conveniences, fast foods, toxic foods, and eating addictions. With chronic Lyme, the body is already stressed, and it is helpful to pay attention to our daily eating habits. We must become aware of what, how, and when we eat and how well we chew our food (or not).

The more you eat home-cooked foods, the better. That way you can control and know what is—or is not—in your food. Avoiding rancid vegetable oils, antibiotics, yeast, chemicals, preservatives, and GMOs in externally prepared food is important. So is the risk of possible exposure to gluten, additives, or MSG, which you might not tolerate. There can also be harmful parasites lurking in your restaurant-ordered sushi, and one is more likely to end up with accidental food poisoning due to inappropriate food storage in warmer months.

Becoming mindful of poor eating habits, such as eating while you watch TV or when checking your iPhone for emails, is very important. These common and addictive habits can influence your chewing, enzyme release, and digestive ability. Instead, put on some soothing music or light a candle. Creating a calm and peaceful environment at mealtimes is part of a daily nourishing strategy.

When living with persistent Lyme, begin your healing path by integrating healthy foods, a regular nourishing schedule, optimal digestion, and gut healing. Think of this book as a jump-start into a nutritional healing strategy that supports your unique biochemistry. (Once you have implemented the foundational action steps that support your digestive and gut health, Metabolic Typing, www.healthexcel.com, is a great way to learn more about your individual dietary needs.)

What we eat supports our blood sugar balance, or it can make us feel tired and cause inflammation. We must eat for vitality, not just for calories. When living with chronic Lyme, the quality of calories matter greatly. Whole, organic foods with phytonutrients, antioxidants, fiber, bioflavonoids, phenols, carotenoids, alkaloids, minerals, and vitamins directly affect our ability to handle tough infections because they support our immune system and energy.

Whole foods encourage healing at a cellular level. The nutrients in whole foods are in dosages that will not overpower the human body, so it is important to eat a diet that is diverse and seasonal. All foods in nature occur as a whole, and it is in this form that the DNA in our cells recognizes nutritional fortification. Foods communicate with your body through your DNA; is that not fascinating? Food has the ability to switch on harmful genes and to keep harmful genes silent. We are now studying how organic foods and phytonutrients in plants have the ability to override our inherited genetic weaknesses, and that is exciting.

The sad part is that our soil, crops, and foods do not have the nutrient value they had over a hundred years ago, and the air pollution and acid rain contaminates organic crops, too. Processing of foods has stripped them of much-needed fiber, and it alters the structure of proteins in foods, creating more food allergies and food intolerances. As a result, malnutrition because of a lack of nutrients, not calories, is a common occurrence.

Your food choices directly influence the diversity of your gut flora, and that makes a difference in your energy, symptoms, and resilience. Our gut flora plays an important role in transforming foods into useable nutrients, which influences our blood sugar levels. Bitter foods, multicolored foods, and naturally sweet foods, to name a few, all have a specific role in communicating to different microbes, organ functions, and mechanical actions in the body.

Let us consider that nourishing also begins with how we eat. Not chewing food properly, until it is more liquefied and broken down into small particles, sets the scene for indigestion. The act of chewing is communication between the brain and the stomach. This stimulates the release of enzymes from the pancreas, the production of hydrochloric acid in the stomach, and the release of bile from the gallbladder.

The digestive process is like a ladder: If you shake it at the top, the turbulence reverberates all the way to the bottom, just like our gut. If our digestion is compromised by our food choices, lack of chewing, and lack of stomach acid, it will eventually lead to challenges in various lower parts of the digestive tract.

Individual digestive weaknesses and challenges must be investigated, whether one is in current treatment for Lyme infections or not. Unexplained weight gain or muscle loss, upset stomach, and abdominal pains can all be—or may not be—related to chronic Lyme infections. Severe, daily, uncomfortable stomach and bowel problems can make you afraid to eat anything. Gall stones and infections can result in pancreatitis, removal of the gallbladder, and additional infections. When taking nutritional supplements, swallowing pills is difficult for some and absorption is often a challenge; thus, supplementation in powder, chewable, sublingual, liposomal, topical, and liquid form is more effective.

Determining how much energy a processed food contains is simple: Take a look at the preservatives listed on the food label and the expiration date on the package. The longer the shelf life listed on the outside of the product, the less nutrient rich the food is on the inside. Consider the life span of an apple. It's only good for a short while after you pick it. Natural foods have a life cycle; however, processed foods do not, and so I call them *nonfoods*. The next time you are in a grocery store, check out the shelf life of some of the products.

Some commercial foods are even labeled *heart healthy*, but this is not so. They are not healthy foods; they are simply well-marketed foods. Commercial foods are stripped of their natural fiber, vitamins, and minerals during processing. This is especially true regarding vitamins A, B, C, E, calcium, magnesium, selenium, and iodine, which our bodies need to strengthen the immune, nervous, and hormonal systems. A fortified food is enhanced with synthetic vitamins, which cannot be, and must not be, compared with complete vitamin complexes found in whole foods.

The body has a challenging time creating vitamin complexes out of synthetically enriched foods, because certain cofactors and enzymes are missing from them. It has to draw on its own (already limited) resources to create a vitamin complex from synthetic, isolated vitamins. This takes a lot of effort on the part of your body, as does getting rid of chemical toxins in foods, such as food coloring or synthetic sweeteners. Does your body have enough energy and the right nutrients to accomplish this? Processed, man-made foods include isolated, heat-treated, synthetic, and fractionated nutrients, which resemble no food in nature. Overconsumption of fortified foods, such as synthetic folic acid, creates biochemical dysfunction in the body.

Iodized salt contains sufficient iodine to prevent goiter formation; however, it is insufficient for the body's overall needs. Recommended dietary allowance (RDA) levels are too vague and generalized, with mostly insufficient recommendations regarding vitamin and mineral levels.

Commercial food products are pasteurized, homogenized, and at times ultrapasteurized—the companies really kill the vitality and damage the nutrients with high heat so it can have a long shelf life. These are not brain and energy-supporting foods; avoid them as best as you can. With excessive heat treatment, the proteins in the foods have been altered, and these can trigger inflammation, food allergies, or sensitivities. The heat also alters the fats and turns them rancid. Chemicals and fragrances are added to cover the rancidity, yet the body is not fooled by these harmful fats that clog up the gallbladder and cell membranes and contribute to systemic inflammation, weight gain, and cholesterol challenges.

Avoid these common toxic commercial foods as much as possible:

- Processed foods
- Nonorganic dairy products
- Fried and fast foods
- All canned food, especially with BPA (bisphenol A) plastic lining

- Foods with *natural flavoring* (This is misleading.)
- Factory farmed beef, pork, and poultry
- Farmed fish with antibiotics, coloring, and growth hormones
- Commercial milk, cottage cheese, nonfat yogurt, processed cheese, commercial butter or butter-like spreads, and commercial eggs
- Any heat-treated oils in clear plastic bottles, including canola oil, vegetable, and sunflower oil
- Frozen dinners with excessive sodium and preservatives
- Syrups, jams, cookies, chocolate, and candy containing GMO high-fructose corn syrup, GMO soybean oil, and trans fats
- GMO soy products
- Nonorganic vegetables and fruits with excessive pesticide and insecticide sprayings that are grown in poor soil
- Ice cream made with artificial colors, added flavors, hormones, or antibiotics and GMO high-fructose corn syrup
- Soda pop and fruit juices (most contain concentrated sugars and are high glycemic)
- Popular mega-calorie coffee drinks with fake cream and sugar-laden syrups

When shopping, stay clear of all nonfat or zero percent fat food products. These contain fillers, gums, and extra sugars to compensate for lack of fat and lack of taste. The body needs healthy fats. There is no food in nature that is a hundred percent fat-free. We need fat to absorb essential vitamins A, D, E, and K; thus, absorption is inhibited in any product that contains zero percent fat. Nonfat foods can irritate and clog up the digestive tract, they create hunger because you are not satiated, and they are a source of empty calories that do not satisfy the body's nutrient needs.

Pasteurized yogurt comes back to life because probiotic cultures are added after the heating process. If dairy is tolerated, raw is best—or find the least pasteurized version possible. If dairy does not agree with you, experiment with a small amount of coconut yogurt and see if your body tolerates that. Coconut products are healthy, but they are not right for everyone. There are various possible reasons for intolerance, including heritage or microbial overgrowth in the gut. There are great online resources regarding homemade kefir or yogurt, which is always preferable to store-bought items.

Refined sugars, soda or diet soda, and concentrated fruit juices quickly spike the blood sugar, which results in a blood sugar crash, creating a craving for more sugar. High-fructose corn syrup is extremely addictive for the brain, and it is highly inflammatory. This processed sweetener creates a turbo boost on blood sugar spikes and continuous pancreatic, adrenal, and liver stress. If you have a sweet tooth or a sugar craving, indulge in a lower glycemic fruit, unsweetened applesauce with stevia, a piece of organic dark chocolate, or a small bowl of coconut yogurt with berries or cinnamon rather than indulging in commercial candy, soda, or multicolored electrolyte drinks with GMO high-fructose corn syrup and artificial ingredients.

Go Organic: GMO Foods, Antibiotic, and Glyphosate

There is great pushback globally against GMO foods. At present, thirty-eight countries worldwide have banned cultivation of GMO foods. African countries are still facing great pressure from Biotech companies and the Gates Foundation to lift bans on GMO unmilled food aid.[1]

GMO foods should be labeled. As consumers, it is our right to know what is in the food we are buying. Here in the United States, after great public support, the Deny Americans the Right to Know (DARK) act that prohibited labeling of GMO foods was not passed in the Senate. However, after much political wrangling, with major food corporations and government lobbyists pushing their deceptive and profit-driven agendas at the expense of our health and our planet, President Obama signed off on the DARK Act in July 2016.

As consumers, we must take a stand with our wallets and support free-range suppliers and local farmers, not industrial factory farms that harm us, animals, oceans, and plant life. Pasture-raised meat and free-range animal products are more expensive, but your body will be able to absorb many more nutrients and healthy fats without being exposed to additional poisons, cancer-promoting growth factors, and more antibiotics. You might not be able to tell the difference between a commercial short-rib, stew, or beef patty and free-range meats, but your body certainly can.

A factory-farmed, disease-ridden, and poorly-fed animal will not improve anyone's health. It is inhumane how animals are raised on feedlots, pumped with hormones, antibiotics, GMO corn, grains, and soy to fatten them up quickly so they reach a certain weight.[2] An estimated eighty percent of all feedlot cattle are injected with hormones or given an ear implant to make them grow faster and to increase milk production. The FDA and USDA claim that these hormones are safe for human consumption, yet the endocrine disruption with accumulative residues of growth hormones in the food chain is well known.[3] This greatly affects children and teenagers before puberty. Scientists, farmers, and consumers opposed rBGH-treated dairy products; however, the FDA approved rBGH after relying on one study done by Monsanto, testing its effects on thirty rats over a course of ninety days. The study was never released. There has never been a full review by the FDA despite warnings and bans of rBGH in Europe and other countries.

The pesticide glyphosate, the active ingredient in the popular weed killer RoundUp from Monsanto, is known to disrupt the metabolism and hormones, cause cancer, and destroy the nervous system and gut in humans, fish, and animals.[4] It also interferes with the metabolism of vitamin D, mineral absorption, and adversely shifts the balance within the microbiome. Glyphosate is associated with severe manganese deficiency, which impacts neurological diseases, osteoporosis, autism, depletion of needed lactobacillus bacteria in the gut, and infertility. It is banned in many countries around the world, but not in the United States.[5]

In 2015, industrial use of glyphosate was listed as "possibly carcinogenic to humans." This created a great uproar from Monsanto because it brought increased attention to the dangers of herbicides and pesticides that are commonplace in our foods. Traces from spraying end up contaminating the air, water, soil, forests, organic farms, and other continents—where glyphosate is banned.

The chronic, low-grade exposure to glyphosate, and all other environmental toxins, adds up in the body. Toxicity is one of the root causes of inflammation; it is implicated in every disease. Even fish develop illness that mimics celiac disease after exposure to glyphosate.[6]

GMO foods transfer antibiotics into our cells in the gut, interfering with the body's immune function. This is known as *horizontal gene transfer,* and it contributes to many digestive and immune disruptions with long-lasting health implications. This also contributes to the rise in antibiotic resistance and cancers.[7]

Because of the many toxins in our food supply, I recommend choosing a diet made up primarily of organic foods. It is much easier to eat this way at home, where you can control the quality and sourcing of your food. When eating out or traveling, you don't have as much control over exposure to GMO and commercially processed foods.

If you are able to have a small vegetable garden by your home, that is great. If you can't, buy local foods and sustainable foods as much as possible. When you are sick, your body needs nutrition from whole foods grown in healthy soil, not more chemicals, high fructose corn syrup, MSG, and toxins.

Should you buy commercial produce or produce that is not locally sourced, wash it well to remove the pesticide poisons as much as possible—and peel the fruit or vegetable (e.g., cucumbers, zucchini, peaches, pears, and apples) because many pesticides are embedded in the skin. When we lose the peel, sadly, we also lose a source of needed fiber that is helpful for stabilizing blood sugar and maintaining healthy gut flora.

Choose foods with the label *USDA-certified organic,* and choose hormone-free and antibiotic-free animal and dairy products. Consider organic produce at the supermarket if you have no access to a local market. Yes, organic foods are contaminated too because of air and rainfall; however, they have neither endured the excessive and repeated sprayings in industrial food production, nor have they been grown from genetically engineered RoundUp-ready seeds that are designed to tolerate high doses of glyphosate.

Traditional Chinese Medicine Perspective and the Properties of Food

We must also consider the food we eat in our healing journey from a Traditional Chinese Medicine (TCM) perspective. Some of this information possibly contradicts what you might be reading in health books or hearing in the media, yet we must consider the wisdom imparted by other traditional healing modalities, including TCM principles. Food is not just about calories and vitamins, it is about energy too.

Whole foods have energetic properties that get transferred to us. Foods affect our body, creating sensations of hot, cold, warm, cool, and neutral. You might have heard of foods as being yin (cooling); they help to clear toxins and heat from the body. Or you might have heard about yang foods that warm the body by increasing circulation and energy. It is at this energetic level that foods can affect our organs, meridians, and glands. Yin foods include various fruits (including watermelon, banana, or apples), watercress, tomato, buckwheat, cauliflower, and egg whites. Yang foods can include onions, asparagus, cinnamon, black pepper, pomegranate, coffee, chicken, walnuts, and more. Neutral foods include sweet potato, carrots, beetroot, apricots, kidney beans, sunflower seeds, shiitake mushrooms, beef, egg yolk, and honey.

By considering the energetic properties of foods, we can incorporate their healing opportunities when living with persistent Lyme. Foods are used to clean, regulate, and tone the body. Depending on your symptoms, foods can play an important role. They can help the body to grow stronger while increasing its resilience, energy, and innate ability to fight off infections.

Weakened immune and digestive systems will benefit from warm or cooked foods, such as lamb, squash, butter, and chicken. These act like an internal furnace by improving circulation in hands and feet, alleviating stomach pains, and increasing energy. With a rash or heat-associated skin problems, eating raw and cooling foods, such as celery, lettuce, fruits, and green leafy vegetables, will decrease the internal heat.

In addition to the energetic properties of foods, flavors of foods influence our health. The five flavors include sweet, sour, bitter, sweet, and pungent, and they affect all the organs in our body.

Sweet foods affect the stomach and spleen. They lubricate and nourish the body. Some examples are sweet potato, pumpkin, peas, rice, honey, dates, shiitake, cucumber, and mushroom. As the immune system is closely connected with the spleen, foods that nourish the spleen are very important because they also support digestion.

With today's diet, our bitter taste buds have been downgraded and our sweet taste has been dramatically upgraded. Our digestion and our body pay the price. We have bitter taste sensors in cells of organs and glands, even on our thyroid, lungs, and in semen in men. This is a taste that is acknowledged in the Ayurvedic and Traditional Chinese Medicine philosophies, yet it is severely neglected in the Standard American Diet. Coffee is a well-known bitter substance. Others are endives, kale, arugula, eggplant, radicchio, dandelion, wormwood, gentian, goldenseal, Swedish bitters, andrographis, bitter melon, and feverfew.

Bitters stimulate digestive secretions, increase appetite when one is underweight and ill, ease a constipated colon, encourage satiety, ease dampness, lower allergic responses, and purge heat in the body during fevers. Bitters register on the tongue and on many cells in the body, including the brain, vagus nerve, and all digestive organs. Taste sensitivity varies greatly in different cultures. Some sensitive individuals have a low tolerance for the bitter taste. It can make them feel nauseous, as they may have a genetic glitch in some of their bitter taste receptors. Generally, it is best to add a warming spice or herb when supplementing with bitters, because bitters innately have a cooling property.

Bitter foods support our immune function. Their compounds are akin to a plant toxin that wakes up the T and B immune cells in the body—the adaptive immune system. In addition, findings show that bitters dial down allergic responses, including mast cell responses that are associated with inflammation, asthma, and various other histamine-related health symptoms. Because of this broad spectrum effect, supplementing with bitters or adding them to your food is a health-supporting necessity when living with chronic Lyme.

Bitter foods affect the heart and the small intestine, clear heat, stimulate the appetite, and promote bowel movements. Bitter foods stimulate the release of bile. This is one reason why Swedish bitters is often recommended to support digestion.

Sour foods affect the liver and gallbladder, which is really important with Lyme infections. Sour foods are an astringent that assists in the elimination of fluids and toxic substances in the body, while also acting like a brake on excessive elimination involving diarrhea and heavy perspiration. Sour foods include lemon, olives, plums, royal jelly, pineapple, and vinegar.

Salty foods affect the kidney and bladder (and the adrenals too). These foods help nourish the blood, break up hardness, lubricate the intestines, and support bowel activity. They include millet, duck meat, shellfish, and bone marrow. Adrenal fatigue and low blood pressure are related to an increased need for minerals and thus can contribute to salt cravings.

Pungent foods affect the lungs and the large intestine. Pungent foods support circulation and promote the appetite. These foods include fresh ginger, onion, leeks, celery, spearmint, turnips, mustard seed, radish leaf, and garlic.

Food Sensitivities

All food sensitivities must be seen in context with current Lyme-related symptoms (and antibiotic use) that greatly disrupt the digestive tract. You might not tolerate certain foods and are already eliminating multiple foods, or maybe you have been experiencing digestive or gallbladder problems for a while. These greatly influence your dietary choices. With persistent Lyme infections, many foods can be inflammatory triggers in a compromised gut.

The challenge with any food sensitivity is that its origins might have been present before the Lyme-related infection, yet the symptoms were occasional or mild compared to today. A leaky gut might have already been present because of gluten, stress, alcohol, and over-the-counter medicine use; however, there were no symptoms besides a few skin problems or occasional bloating and burping. And it got better.

Lyme-related infections in the gut can suppress the immune system, allowing secondary infections to occur; or they may instigate an overreactive immune response with molecular mimicry, resulting in autoimmune conditions in the gut in which your own tissues get attacked. This dysregulation invites inflammation and a breakdown of the protective mucosal lining in the gut, which contributes to food sensitivities—and food sensitivities complicate the Lyme scenario. Just like a wristwatch, all moving parts matter; everything works together.

Foods can help or harm us, and it is different for each individual. When it comes to optimal food choices, it is tricky in many cases; some individuals can eat most anything without a problem, and others cannot tolerate many foods at all.

My clients with chronic Lyme have displayed multiple food sensitivities, indigestion, burping, bloating, reflux, headaches, and more, which severely limits their initial food choices.

Yeast, dairy, foods with high histamine levels, such as avocado, and other food that you might have tolerated in the past are possibly creating additional problems for you today. When it comes to the daily diet, the following two points are very important:

- It is not about the foods, it is about how your body responds to the foods.
- It is not about the foods, it is about the health of your gut and the tolerance of your gut immune system.

The so-called *white* foods (processed foods containing white flour, excessive refined salt, and refined sugar) are toxic for everyone. Known inflammatory foods include gluten, sugar, dairy, corn, soy, nuts, chocolate, tomatoes, potatoes, eggplant, peppers, spinach, and citrus fruits. It is the cumulative load of repetitive food triggers that can bring on sensitivities; however, small amounts might be (or might have been) tolerated. It is best to focus on a variety of whole foods, including colorful vegetables and fruits. Preparing foods at home is one way to ward off exposure to spoiled foods, preservatives, and food additives that are also inflammatory triggers.

Factors Impacting Food Sensitivities and a Leaky Gut

- Vector-borne infections
- The quality of foods that you eat
- How frequently a food is consumed
- Food irritants such as gluten or dairy

- Genetic factors
- Adrenal status
- Altered gut flora
- Emotional trauma, physical trauma, or injury
- Celiac disease
- Hidden gut infections (e.g. *Giardia, Cryptosporidium,* and worms)

There are many different dietary options available; you must find the one that best fits your needs and tolerances. Some have already tried a raw food diet or a ketogenic diet or a Paleo diet. The ketogenic and Paleo diets are high in fat and protein and low in carbohydrates. While they may work for many individuals, others do not tolerate those dietary approaches at all. Some individuals do well with juicing, others do not. Certain foods, such as broccoli, tomatoes, fermented sauerkraut, or goat milk yogurt, can be very health supporting; however, for some individuals, they can also cause digestive, joint, or skin problems, in addition to increased brain fog and other debilitating symptoms.

Hidden infections in the gut can cause intolerance of high-fiber foods, and severe dietary modifications are often necessary; they can also mimic Lyme infections that target the gut, including *Bartonella,* resulting in the suppression of the gut's immune system, or they can also mimic symptoms of an autoimmune disease. With use of antibiotics, digestive troubles, and vector-borne infections advanced lab testing is essential.

Food sensitivities are part of the digestive labyrinth. From my experience, multiple food sensitivities are often present in chronically ill individuals, and that can make food rotation more difficult to navigate in the initial stages. Simple starches such as potatoes and white rice are often tolerated, yet these foods create blood sugar spikes and feed fungal infections. I have worked with a client who initially could barely tolerate five foods. Yes, *five foods!*

Advanced food sensitivity testing is not always an option, so consider some do-it-yourself options.

KEEP A DETAILED FOOD DIARY TO TRACK
DAILY FOOD INTAKE AND SYMPTOMS.

To learn more about your specific digestive ailments and a possible food correlation, it is best to keep a food diary and to track your symptoms. I ask all my clients for a four-day food diary before meeting with me. These provide a wealth of information that include blood sugar slumps and food comas after meals. Could there be a connection with the foods you are eating and your symptoms, even if you are eating healthy organic foods?

For one week, keep notes on all the foods and drinks you consume, including time of consumption. Track if or how soon digestive ailments, energy slumps, sleep quality, increased pain, mood swings, or mental sluggishness appear after eating. It is not always easy, I know, to keep a diary of your diet, but make it a priority. And be aware that symptoms might appear soon after eating, but delayed reactions to foods can be up to seventy-two hours later.

AN ELIMINATION DIET OR FOOD CHALLENGE IS A SELF-TEST
THAT ALLOWS YOU TO EAVESDROP ON YOUR BODY.

If you do not know which foods you are sensitive to, consider an inexpensive and effective self-test. For three weeks, eliminate inflammatory foods from your diet and keep track of any digestive changes or easing of symptoms in a food diary. After the three-week period, you can reintroduce these foods, one by one.

An easy way to get started on any basic elimination diet is by eliminating the common inflammatory culprits; take out either gluten or dairy first. Eggs can be problematic too, so eliminate them if you choose to eliminate dairy. See if symptoms improve. You may experience less bloating and gas or skin changes. Notice if you feel more focused, you sleep a little better, or your blood sugar does not crash after eating a meal when you eliminate these foods.

If you are feeling an obvious change for the better—good. After three weeks, eat a lot of the food group you eliminated and see how your digestion and pain symptoms are affected. If prior symptoms return with a vengeance, because the immune system is provoked after abstinence, you will know those are offenders.

Below are the top five most common food allergens that contribute to inflammation and an overactive immune response in the body:

- Gluten
- Corn
- Soy
- Dairy (excluding butter and eggs)
- Nuts

If you are already eliminating the top five culprits, refer to chapter seven for more food triggers that might be causing your problems. For example, you could eliminate cruciferous vegetables or citrus fruits for a therapeutic time frame and see if that eases symptoms. Take note of any changes and improvements in your digestive symptoms by eliminating that particular group of vegetables or fruits, which can be difficult to digest.

Consider that you might be having digestive troubles because of digestive insufficiencies—not because of a food intolerance. You might be eating healthy, but insufficient hydrochloric acid in the stomach will restrict digestive power. This can lead to constipation and bloating or acid reflux, which mimic a food sensitivity. Drinking raw apple cider vinegar with water ten to fifteen minutes before meals is very helpful.

If you are on an acid-blocking medication, it will impact mineral absorption, and you might experience more cramping and spasms in your lower legs during the night or cavities in your teeth. Zinc, a very important mineral for the immune system, is required for hydrochloric acid production, and we need hydrochloric acid to absorb zinc—it really can be a vicious cycle!

FODMAPS: Why Certain Carbohydrates Might Not Be Good For You

High fiber vegetables can be troublesome for some after prolonged antibiotic treatment, when Lyme infections or Bell's palsy affect the gut flora, or when constipated. High-fiber vegetables, especially of the allium, cruciferous, or brassica varieties, are known as FODMAP foods (fermentable oligosaccharides, disaccharides, monosaccharides, and polyols). When bacterial overgrowth and slow transit time are present, the fiber and sugar in these FODMAP foods can be fermented by bacteria that have migrated from the bowels into the small intestine;

this contributes to uncomfortable and often embarrassing symptoms including gas, bloating, burping, laxity in the esophageal sphincter, and acid reflux.

Antibiotic use is one of the root causes for this bacterial overgrowth; however, there can be many other root causes, such as Lyme infections and prior unresolved food poisonings. This infection is tenacious, and required dietary modifications are different for everyone. It is often diagnosed, or not, as small intestinal bacterial overgrowth (SIBO) with a breath test in a doctor's office.

SIBO can also be a side effect of medications affecting the diversity of the microbiome (gut ecology), or it can be caused by damaged nerves in the intestinal wall, inhibiting a natural clearing action. When this happens, food waste hangs on and is not eliminated, allowing opportunistic bacteria to migrate and propagate, especially when the immune system is challenged already. *It is not necessarily the Lyme. . . . but Lyme can cause SIBO.*

Relief can occur when offending high-fiber vegetables and fruits are omitted or severely restricted. You might be able to tolerate some high FODMAP foods or only a little, and eating too much of these might cause abdominal discomfort anyway. Every case is different. Low FODMAP foods include all proteins, healthy oils, butter and eggs, fruits (including papaya, kiwi, strawberries, and cranberries), and low-fiber vegetables (including butternut squash, carrots, cucumber, lettuce, and parsnips). There are various lists available online; a great starting point is siboinfo.com.

SIBO must be treated before tolerance of high-fiber vegetables can occur. It takes time, especially when Lyme infections are in play; severe antibiotic treatment is in most cases not an option and not tolerated by the individual with SIBO, and relapses can occur. Therapeutic herbal and homeopathic therapies are effective, but dosages must be titrated up slowly to avoid a herx reaction or a Lyme flare. Finding the right treatment can take many months with these stubborn infections. For more details, see chapter seven.

Plant, Fruit, Seed, and Grain Toxins

Plants provide a source of energy and the phytonutrients are healing to the body. We need plants in our daily diet to be well, and they have the healing potential to keep harmful genes switched off. However, plants have innate defense systems in the form of toxins to ensure their survival against predators in nature; these toxins can be inflammatory for our bodies.

Four key innate plant toxins include—

1   Phytic acid in grains, plants, legumes, nuts, and seeds
2   Oxalates in fruits and vegetables
3   Lectins in legumes and vegetables
4   Goitrogens in legumes, brassicae, and cruciferous vegetables

Grains, nuts, seeds, and legumes produce phytic acid—their natural defense against early sprouting. We often do not have the digestive power to break down these substances, or we might be sensitive to the proteins.

Oxalates in vegetables and fruits vary because the climate, nutrients in the soil, and ripeness differ when eaten. High-oxalate foods include beetroot, soy products, sweet potatoes, spinach, figs, rhubarb, lentils, buckwheat, and chocolate. Paying attention to serving size and food preparation is important because you might be able to tolerate medium- and low-grade oxalate foods. Oxalates create small crystals that can cause joint pain. These are also implicated in kidney stones, gout, vulvodynia, interstitial cystitis, and joint pain in the extremities. High oxalate levels are also implicated in mental and behavioral challenges, especially in children with autism. A key component is a lack of oxalate-degrading bacteria in the gut, called *Oxalobacter formigenes*, which is diminished by the use of antibiotics. Scientific and clinical research is ongoing in this arena.

Goitrogens inhibit the absorption of important minerals such as calcium, magnesium, zinc, and B12, and they can also inhibit thyroid function. With sluggish digestion, consumption of raw vegetables can be challenging. Yes, there are other plant toxins and phytochemicals that can create digestive or inflammatory challenges; however, the ones mentioned in this chapter are our main considerations at this time.

Cook, steam, or sauté all dark leafy greens to neutralize oxalic acid, goitrogens, lectins, and phytic acid that bind to much-needed minerals, such as calcium, magnesium, and zinc, and that inhibit mineral and vitamin absorption. This is one good reason not to eat raw spinach, kale, or nuts. Eating a colorful, plant-based, whole food diet is part of our goal, but digesting and absorbing the nutrients in foods is what we are really after. To support yourself in that goal, food preparation is crucial, especially when dealing with chronic fatigue. Ironically, this food prep is more work for those who are already so tired, but it goes a long way.

A SPECIAL NOTE ON FOLIC ACID AND FOLATE

You do not want to confuse folate with the synthetic folic acid that is used to fortify processed foods. The government ordered the mandatory folic acid fortification of many commercial foods in 1998. It was a protective measure against neural tube defects. But now, with the overconsumption of processed foods, many end up having too much in their systems. This adds liver stress because excess folic acid cannot be converted into bioavailable folate.[8]

Elevated synthetic folic acid has been associated with an increased risk of cancer.[9] It can also mask a vitamin B12 deficiency, which is associated with multiple symptoms, especially cognition, heart, and neurological disorders.

Folic acid is also found in processed foods and in nutritional supplements. Many individuals cannot metabolize the synthetic folic acid into a bioavailable form, and it builds up in the bloodstream instead of being transported into the cells, which need it to function well.

Think big picture—*your* big picture. To start, complete the following exercise:

Healthy Eating Deposit

» Check off the actions you will commit to taking today

- ☐ Eat three to four different organic, brightly colored vegetables and one fruit. Count and keep a list of the various colors you eat every day.
- ☐ Eat a whole food breakfast within one hour of waking. Include sources of protein, fat, and carbohydrate. (Fruit is a carb.)
- ☐ Cut out of gluten-containing foods: barley, rye, oats, wheat, and spelt.

☐ Plan a weekly home-cooked meal. Prepare a shopping list.

☐ Sit down while eating your meals. Take time to chew your food thoroughly with a sense of gratitude. Appreciate the flavors and textures of foods.

☐ Start using a probiotic from a reputable company to support gut flora balance and diversity.

☐ Add fermented vegetables as a condiment three to four times per week to promote gut flora wellness (not with certain gut problems).

☐ Each time you shop, buy two to three different colored vegetables. Always include a dark green vegetable. (Organic is best.)

☐ Cut out daily diet soda and commercial fruit juices. Instead, drink a few glasses of water throughout the day or include some caffeine-free herbal tea.

☐ Get rid of cooking oils in white plastic bottles in your kitchen. Only use olive oil in dark green bottles and organic butter, plant, and seed oils in glass bottles.

☐ Start your day with a glass of water with lemon juice.

☐ Sign up for the Advanced Metabolic Typing Test (online test).

· · · · · · ·

Wrapping Up

The life force, the prana or chi, is contained in a large variety of soil-grown, pasture-raised, and ocean-living whole foods that provide our bodies with much-needed energy, nourishment, and resilience. How do the foods that you consume daily support your life force? Sure, on some days you will not be able to eat organic foods, but think about the implication of how your daily eating habits influence your ability to have more energy during the day and to fight infections. Foods can harm or heal depending on the individual; this is why there is no one-size-fits-all approach.

Avoiding foods that irritate and burden the body is the first line of defense for decreasing inflammation on a localized and systemic level. Another helpful practice is food rotation, or rotating the foods that you eat every four days. This gives the gut's immune system time to calm itself, in case it was irritated by one of the consumed foods.

Getting rid of hidden infections and rebalancing gut flora is the second line of defense. With complex cases, it is best to consult with a knowledgeable nutritional clinician to determine a customized nutritional strategy and protocol for gut healing. You have the power to bring life force and energy into your body through the foods that you consume every day. No medication can do that for you, even if your physician, endocrinologist, or psychiatrist thinks it can.

"Don't eat anything your great-great grandmother wouldn't recognize as food. There are a great many food-like items in the supermarket your ancestors wouldn't recognize as food. . . . stay away from these."

—MICHAEL POLLAN

Chapter Four

The Whole Food Kaleidoscope

It is essential to focus on nutrient-dense whole foods when living with a chronic illness. Certain food choices might be deemed healthy, yet they are inappropriate for you. With that in mind, you will be able to make better choices for your daily nourishment. Let us now discuss food choices that contribute to the whole food kaleidoscope.

Simple and Complex Carbohydrates

Carbohydrates provide us with vitamins, nutrients, fiber, and the energy needed to digest protein and fats in food. We need carbohydrates for blood sugar control, but not refined and processed sugars that induce roller-coaster blood sugar spikes and dips, lack of focus, mood swings, and fatigue.

We need carbohydrates to raise our blood sugar. How much or how little and which type is best tolerated requires fine-tuning based on the individual's biochemistry, stress levels, and overall health. For some, a small amount of a starchy vegetable or grain that is buffered with free-range animal proteins and fats is well tolerated, while others do better with some seasonal fruit, complex carbohydrate vegetables, and lighter proteins and oils.

Consumption of carbohydrates plays an important role in sustaining our energy throughout the day and night. When living with Lyme, it is best to choose more complex carbohydrates and to buffer them with a source of protein and fat.

This offsets the erratic blood sugar imbalances associated with chronic infections and adrenal insufficiency.

Eating too many starches or sugary carbs with any snack or meal will spike blood sugar and stress our pancreas, adrenals, and liver; this contributes to weight gain as insulin converts excess sugars into stored fat. Small things like drinking a glass of processed orange juice, eating a slice of toast with jam, drinking coffee without the buffer of a meal, noshing on a handful of raisins or jellybeans, or enjoying a pineapple and strawberry nonfat smoothie will contribute to blood sugar swings. However, eating too few carbs is a concern too because it can trigger a hypoglycemic episode, which is also interconnected with low cortisol output from the adrenal glands. We want to use foods, not tired adrenals, to raise and stabilize our blood sugar during the day.

When our energy is low, we crave sugar or starchy carbohydrates. Our brain is experiencing an energy crisis and needs a source of sugar fast, and carbohydrates equal quick energy. If we skip meals, do not eat enough calories, or are in a hypoglycemic episode, the body will use stored glycogen in the liver for brain energy. That supply is limited. Our muscles become an emergency reservoir of energy the body uses to sustain vital bodily functions when the body is in crisis, or when we are very ill.

THE COMPLEXITIES OF COMPLEX CARBOHYDRATES

Complex carbohydrates, such as celery, cucumber, cabbages, cauliflower, broccoli, brussels sprouts, or dandelions, are great carbohydrate options when blood sugar problems are present. Besides adding color to your plate, these vegetables are nutrient-rich, cancer protective, lower in sugar, and high in fiber, especially when grown in healthy organic soil. Lower-glycemic carbs, such as complex carbohydrate vegetables (and some legumes), sufficiently maintain a stable level of blood sugar for three to four hours. The fiber in these foods offsets hypoglycemia, which is associated with simple, processed sugars and starchy foods.

Legumes, including beans, peas, and lentils, are a combination of complex and starchy carbohydrates; they are a great source of protein, magnesium, B vitamins, copper, and insoluble fiber. With severe blood sugar swings, I do recommend pairing legumes with a low-glycemic vegetable and adding a protein and fat source.

Prepare legumes, including lentils, peas, and kidney, navy, pinto, adzuki, mung, and lima beans, well to maximize nutrient absorption. It is best to soak and drain them, then cook them sufficiently to neutralize the thyroid-inhibiting phytic acid and lectins. Organic canned beans can be a quick, easy, go-to option. Cook and strain the canned beans well to make them easier to digest, even though they are precooked.

Vegetables that are high in bioavailable folate include leafy greens like Swiss chard, dandelion, mustard greens, watercress, escarole, spinach, asparagus, parsley, lentils, turnip greens, romaine lettuce, and collard greens. Incidentally, there is phytic acid in spinach and Swiss chard too—another reason to avoid eating raw spinach. (Of note: Free-range calf and chicken livers are the richest sources of folate.)

Plant-based foods are optimal carb choices that support blood cleansing and blood building. They provide bioavailable sources of folate, the water-soluble vitamin B9, which is especially required for detoxification pathways during pregnancy, and DNA protection in the body.

If you live in a warm climate, juicing low-glycemic vegetables and cooling fruits is a nutritional dietary option. Be sure to blanch the vegetables before you juice them, especially dark leafy greens, because juicing of raw vegetables can be tough on a digestive system that is already compromised from antibiotic use. However, just because juicing is touted as being healthy or helpful for someone else, do not assume that will be the case for you; it might not be right for you at this time. Listen to your body.

STARCHY CARBS

We require whole food carbohydrates from various sources; these can include starchy or high-fiber vegetables, fruits, and whole grains. (There are gluten-free grains, including quinoa, sorghum, and amaranth.) These foods are caution foods for some individuals, as they spike blood sugar levels if not appropriately opposed by complex carbs, fats, and protein. With prediabetic or diabetic considerations, check your blood sugar response with a glucometer and make appropriate modifications in your food choices.

Starchy foods that are higher in fiber, such as sweet potatoes, cassava, or plantains, play a very important role in our body. Microbes in the intestines ferment the fiber in these foods, creating butyrate and short-chain fatty acids (SCFA). These have many important functions in the body, including lowering inflammation, calming an overactive immune system, helping a leaky gut heal, affecting the nervous system in the gut, protecting the brain, and aiding in lowering insulin resistance.

Short-chain fatty acids are also infection fighters, which is important in vector-borne and viral infections. With any inflammation or infection in the gut, the production of butyrate is compromised, with far-reaching consequences. This was researched in studies that examined ulcerative colitis, post-infectious irritable bowel syndrome (IBS), and colitis. Colonics with butyrate might be considered as this is a direct delivery route into the colon.[1]

Root and vine growing vegetables such as beets, potatoes, carrots, yams or sweet potatoes, turnips, yucca, and cassava are higher in naturally occurring sugars, yet they have immense health benefits; they contain carotenoids and vitamins and minerals that support our health. Orange, yellow, and red cultured foods are abundant in beta-carotene that can be converted into vitamin A; however, some individuals are not able to do the intrinsic conversion and thus do better with a formed vitamin A, as in cod liver oil. Do eat the beet tops, too, because they reduce gallbladder congestion by thinning the bile. *Optimizing bile flow is very important when dealing with Lyme infections and any therapeutic treatment.*

Root vegetables are also known as warming foods that support digestion and the adrenals. With their sweetness, they satisfy a sweet tooth; they also satisfy the brain and relieve emotional stress. These foods support our energy: Think of a root vegetable like a storage reservoir of energy that will give you energy but include healthy fats and protein to anchor your blood sugar. An example is the combination of a steamed yam combined with bone broth and sea salt in a blender.

Make sure the root vegetables are firm, with fresh leaves and without blemishes, when you buy them at the market or grocery store. It is best to only buy organic because of the lack of nutrients and excessive pesticide sprayings in commercial produce.

GRAINY THOUGHTS

Traditionally, prepared grains are a great source of fiber that supports bowel activity. They are also a source of B vitamins and essential minerals. If the gut is not well, digestion is weak, and if certain genetics are in play, grains can be extremely troublesome and are best eliminated from the present diet.

Whole grains, including whole grain rice, sprouted grains, and cooked breakfast cereals, are a part of many traditional diets. Individuals of European, South American, and Asian descent have a better tolerance for grains. The nutrients and fiber are health supporting. They also play an important role in the bifidia bacteria in our gut flora. Long-term elimination of grains in the diet has been shown to reduce health-supporting gut bacteria. It is important to consider how eliminating grains, or any food group, from your diet affects the microflora in the long term.

Many people cannot tolerate grains. Eating processed grains contributes to additional inflammation, leaky gut, food sensitivities, additional infections, and brain inflammation. But is it the grains, addition of yeasts, or the processing, hybridization, and excessive use of pesticides that are driving the intolerances? Do pesticides harm our gut lining and irritate the immune system so we do not tolerate grains? In addition, selective breeding and processing have altered the structure of traditional grains.

If you tolerate grains, food preparation is important, especially with weakened digestion. Purchase organic grains, look for the stone-ground ones, and store them in a cool place. It is best to buy organic whole grains in small quantities, because the oils in the grains go rancid over time.

When cooking with organic whole grains, soak them in water overnight. Before cooking, rinse the grain and finish preparation with fresh water; also make sure to rinse them well after cooking. Add a pinch of sea salt if so desired, bring them to a boil, and then lower the temperature. Add a lid to the pot and let them simmer until all the liquid is absorbed, without stirring. Once you remove the pot from heat, allow the pot to stand for ten minutes before serving. This is a good way to make some extra for leftovers. Store them in a covered dish in the fridge to use as a ready addition for your soup or as a side dish with your protein and fat.

THE GLUTEN FACTOR

Most patients with Lyme who come to see me have already eliminated gluten from their diets because it was giving them digestive troubles or simply made them feel worse. Gluten increases the severity of Lyme-related symptoms, such as joint pain, brain fog, and bloating. Gluten-containing grains include barley, rye, wheat, and spelt. Oats are gluten free; however, they can be cross contaminated if processed with machinery that also processes gluten-containing foods.

Gluten triggers an inflammatory overreaction from the immune system that is connected with spikes in blood sugar. The inflammation damages the villi, which are finger-like structures that absorb nutrients in the small intestine. Gluten, from the Latin word for glue, also contributes to Lyme-related joint pain, brain inflammation, and other localized or systemic autoimmune symptoms.

When feeling exhausted and depressed, it is easy to become addicted to starchy carbs, including bread, muffins, or cereal. These actually affect brain chemicals, making us feel better for the short term, but they irritate and inflame the body and brain.

Gluten has addictive, drug-like qualities. It converts into morphine-like substances called *gluteomorphins* in the brain, shutting it down while providing a dopamine boost—the feel-good factor. Eliminating gluten can be a challenge because of this addictive effect. Even when eliminating foods that contain gluten, many individuals maintain a carbohydrate addiction with gluten-free foods. Undigested milk proteins, called *casomorphins*, have the same effect on the brain. With any cognitive, behavior, learning disability, and neurological concerns, it is best to avoid gluten-containing foods and dairy.

The Standard American Diet includes a large amount of highly-processed, gluten-containing foods (and sugar). Gluten is often hidden in prepared foods, such as in salad dressings, ice cream, and soy sauce. Beware of the words *natural flavoring* on food labels as well. Check the celiac.com website for more information regarding hidden sources of gluten in foods.

Some individuals might tolerate gluten-containing foods abroad, but the excessive pesticides and herbicides that are sprayed on the crops in the United States cause digestive disturbances and a hypervigilant immune response. Gluten-containing foods are best avoided in the United States because of the constant, low-grade exposure to excessive toxins, especially glyphosate, that are implicated in inflammatory conditions and genetic mutations.

Our gut milieu is more compromised than ever by commercial foods that contain antibiotics, hormones, and chemicals; stress; medications; excessive childhood vaccinations; and rampant environmental pollutants in the soil, water, air, and living environment.

All these factors contribute to a perfect storm for multiple food sensitivities, with gluten often being a final trigger or contributor, because it directly affects the integrity of the gut lining. If the gut is in trouble, we are in trouble. This is still not accepted in commercial medicine, neurology, and psychiatrics, and yet the scientific evidence supporting it is pervasive.[2]

Genetics play an important part in gut health, especially when a genetic factor such as undiagnosed celiac disease is in play. This is a multisystemic disorder, and it does not just affect the gut. One might have a genetic predisposition for celiac disease, but it remains dormant for many years, until health problems present themselves. Non-celiac gluten sensitivity is rapidly on the increase, and it is linked to autoimmune diseases, psychiatric illness, attention deficit hyperactivity disorders, and other behavior problems.

Generally, I do not recommend the popular foods labeled gluten free (GF) in grocery stores, even if they are organic. These often contain a combination of flours, thickeners, and gums, which are produced in a bacterial medium that can include corn, soy, dairy, or wheat, along with yeast, various syrups, and sugars. All have great potential to irritate the immune system, even though they are gluten free. If you are sensitive to just one ingredient, it can cause gut trouble and inflammation.

If you are intolerant of gluten, I recommend baking at home with an alternative ingredient such as coconut flour or almond flour. There are many Paleo recipes online, which you can then customize according to what your body can tolerate—but watch out, some are loaded with natural sugar.

It is best to eliminate or restrict gluten-containing foods when afflicted with the following:

- Vector-borne infections
- Neurological symptoms and diseases
- Chronic digestive disorders
- Chronic joint pain
- Celiac disease
- Hormonal imbalances (including insulin sensitivity, PCOS, and diabetes)
- Skin problems and seasonal allergies
- Auto-immune conditions including rheumatoid arthritis and Hashimoto's thyroiditis

Grains that are gluten-free include amaranth, quinoa, rice, corn, teff, sorghum, Montina Indian ricegrass, buckwheat, and millet. However, cross contamination can occur, so eat these with caution if you are currently having trouble with digestion, joint pain, and cognition.

With nausea during Lyme treatment, eating some tolerated whole grains cooked with fresh ginger, sea salt, and coconut oil will support energy during therapeutic treatment (creamed buckwheat, rice porridge, or starchy vegetables, for instance). These must be balanced with easily digested oils and protein (such as broth or in a chicken soup) to support unstable blood sugar balance associated with chronic Lyme. Coconut or olive oil are best tolerated in these specific circumstances because the liver is stressed and cannot be burdened with heavy fats. On days with severe abdominal pain and relentless nausea, bone or meat broth is helpful for sustenance.

THE FRUITY DILEMMA

Fruits in all colors are a great source of bioflavonoids, carotenoids and antioxidants. They also add some sweetness to a meal and seasonal fruits have always been part of traditional diets during summer months. The skin and the flesh of the fruit offer a good source of fiber; yet it might be best to only consume stewed or baked fruit without the peel when digestive challenges are in play. Fiber in fruit lowers the blood sugar impact from the sugar it contains.

If tolerated, I recommend only eating fruit that is in season, buying it locally, and going organic. The naturally occurring sugar in fruit is called *fructose*, and high sugar fruits are a concern with inflammation, joint pain, gout, and insulin resistance. Apples, berries, cranberries, lemons, and less-ripe pears are lower in naturally occurring sugars; grapes, mangoes, sweet cherries, ripe pears, bananas, pineapple, and kiwi are higher in sugar.

The fruits you buy at the farmer's market have no food label or expiration date, and that is a good sign. Buy organic fruit fresh or frozen, but check that the frozen foods do not contain added sugars, citric acid, or preservatives; these can irritate your gut and brain.

Fruit can spike the blood sugar, so it is best to stay away from all fruit juices, syrups, and all fruit concentrates—even if organic. Yeast and fungal infections in the body love sugar in any form, and in those cases, it is better to eat lower-glycemic fruits such as berries, crisp apples, less-ripe pears, and greenish bananas. The more ripe the fruit, the higher the sugar and histamine content.

Carbs: The Top Three Takeaways

1 Carbs must be balanced with a protein and fat source to support blood sugar balance.

2 Optimize nutrient absorption from vegetables with ideal food preparation, and add bitter foods to support your digestion.

3 We need high fiber carbohydrates to lower inflammation, protect our gut, and move the bowels.

The Power of Protein

We require a variety of proteins as building blocks for our enzymes, hormones, brain chemicals, muscles, bones, organs, and other connective tissues as well as for our detox ability. If you have tooth cavities or bone health challenges, you might want to consider that you are having difficulty absorbing minerals—and protein. Long-term use of acid-blocking medication adds additional complications.

Any type of indigestion and drug therapy will contribute to protein and mineral malabsorption, and this lack of nutrient availability can affect your brain and physical health; you cannot build muscle, repair joints, or rebuild bones without the raw materials known as *amino acids* from the protein we consume. It is all about digestion and absorption.

Animal and other proteins can be difficult to assimilate when digestion has been impaired by lack of stomach acid, chronic use of medications, stress, Lyme-associated infections, gastroparesis, and Bell's palsy-like symptoms in the gut. Appropriate food preparation is key and can include meat broths, ground meats, and pureed fish in more extreme cases. Absorption can also be hampered by tooth or gum problems that limit chewing, imbalances in gut flora, and neurological challenges, including Bell's palsy in the face, when it is difficult to chew foods. Food sensitivities can severely limit protein choices. For example, an individual may rely on eggs, beef, or almond butter as an easy protein choice, yet eggs and peanut butter might not be optimal for that particular individual. (Individuals with a blood type O are more susceptible). Protein deficiencies can show up in muscle loss, depression, blood sugar problems, or in objective findings, such as in a lab test.

There are many types of proteins available. Proteins from animal sources are known as complete proteins, because they contain all the essential and non-essential amino acids. Sources can include broth from marrow bones or chicken bones, wild fish, various cuts of meats, as well as salmon, lamb, free-range eggs, or kefir. Plant proteins, except for soy and quinoa, are not complete proteins. By eating a combination of plant proteins, it is possible to meet the daily requirements of essential amino acids. It is best to tune in to what your body can handle best at this time and what makes you feel well.

Proteins are comprised of various combinations of amino acids that play critical roles in the building and maintenance of organs, glands, enzymes, and other important structures in the body. There are over twenty known amino acids, and they are involved in every function in the body. Their configurations and specific shapes determine their function. They can be part of connective or structural tissues such as the skin, bone, or muscle, they can become a hormone, or they may become brain chemicals, called *neurotransmitters* that affect moods and sleep. The are three categories:

1.   Essential amino acids: They can only be obtained from foods. There are nine essential amino acids—valine, isoleucine, leucine, lysine, methionine, phenylalanine, threonine, histidine, and tryptophan. The body cannot store these amino acids, so our diet must supply them in adequate amounts on a regular basis.

2.   Nonessential amino acids: Your body can create these amino acids from available sources in the body, but their production is provisional. You can only make them if you have enough building materials in your body, and that is often not the case with a deficient diet, challenged digestion, and chronic Lyme. The four amino acids considered nonessential are glutamate, cysteine, asparatate, and alanine.

3.   Conditional, or semi-essential, amino acids include arginine, asparagine, glutamine, tyrosine, glycine, proline, and serine. These are part of the nonessential amino acids that the body can manufacture internally. Even though these amino acids are called nonessential, they perform important roles in the body. Yet, when the body has been under stress for some time and nutrient absorption is insufficient, there is often an underlying amino acid deficiency because the body's nutritional reserves are compromised.

Here's a self-help tip: Drink a glass of water with a half teaspoon of raw apple cider vinegar (Bragg's) ten to fifteen minutes before you eat. If you can tolerate that, increase the apple cider vinegar gradually and carefully to a stronger solution. This will support pH balance and positively affect protein digestion and absorption. (Do not try this with gastric or esophageal inflammation, acid reflux, or the presence of an ulcer. Seek out a health-care professional for guidance.)

WHY PROTEIN MATTERS WHEN LIVING WITH CHRONIC LYME

Eating a protein-dense diet is especially important because the toxic burden from the infections and our environment increase the need for a powerful antioxidant called *glutathione* (GSH). This super antioxidant requires protein in the form of three amino acids (cysteine, glycine, and glutamic acid) for its synthesis inside the body. Think of GSH as a sponge that "sucks up" toxic substances and poisons. In-office IV therapy with glutathione can be part of a medically supervised heavy metal chelation program and Lyme treatment protocol.

With chronic Lyme and coinfections, low levels of GSH make it more difficult to handle the toxic burden from the infections and any antibiotic treatment. (Glutathione levels can be checked with a blood test.) Low GSH levels will also increase your fatigue, brain fog, and overall symptoms of a sluggish metabolism. Glutathione stores become more and more depleted when the body is attempting to prevent the spread of the infection, and trying to take care of collateral damage from the infection or medical interventions.

Glutathione is needed for the immune system and to lower inflammation when chronic infections are present, yet it is most often low in chronically ill individuals, including those with cancer. Proteins become the building blocks for this mega-important detoxing agent. Various vitamins, especially the vitamin B family and vitamin C, and minerals, such as selenium and magnesium, play an important role in the internal recycling of glutathione.

Medications, including antibiotics and pain medications, adversely affect internal production and recycling of GSH. Please note that acetaminophen, antiseizure medications, birth control pills, and antidepressant medications also deplete the body's glutathione stores.

GHS is anti-inflammatory, and a key factor in the elimination of poisons from infections, heavy metals, chemical estrogens in plastics, environmental toxins, and medical drug treatments. If you are having herxing issues when you are in Lyme treatment or are taking antimicrobial herbals, you might consider that a lack of GSH is in play. In supplement form, N-acetyl cysteine (NAC), glycine, and alpha lipoic acid support GSH production and recycling. (Caution: Beware of a possible herx if you are sensitive.)

Whole food sources for GSH production and recycling include animal meats (foods), liver, eggs, dairy, and a quality whey protein shake (if dairy is tolerated). From a plant-based perspective, legumes are also good sources for supporting the GSH pathways as are sulfur foods, including cruciferous vegetables, and the allium family, such as garlic.

An organic whole food whey protein shake is a great source for building blocks of GSH; however, with dairy often not being tolerated, it is not an option for many. If you tolerate whey protein, choose an undenatured, high-quality product. (I use Whey Pro Complete from Standard Process, which contains colostrum and inulin for gastrointestinal immune system support.)

OPTIMAL PROTEIN SOURCES: PASTURE-RAISED ANIMAL FOODS

Proteins from pasture-raised animals are nutrient dense, and they are generally tolerated well by most individuals dealing with Lyme and coinfections. Sometimes various animal proteins are best introduced separately and in small portions because they take energy to digest.

When you buy grass-fed meat, inquire if there was any "finishing off" when the livestock was given grains in their feed. This is cost-effective and occurs in the few months before the animal's last day on earth. It is a common occurrence with larger food chains and in areas where there is a shortage of grazing fields and long winters. "Finishing off" changes the quality of the meat by altering the fatty acid and caloric profile, and it includes more fat.

Pasture-raised animal protein sources include fresh or frozen beef, veal, lamb, poultry, goat, and bison. I always recommend consuming various cuts of the animal and not just consuming the muscle meat. If you do not like heavy proteins and red meat, then listen to your body. You might do better with lighter proteins.

Animal proteins provide bioavailable sources of vitamins A, D, E, and K, zinc, cholesterol, iron, calcium, selenium, and essential fatty acids. These are power foods that can help the body when it is fatigued and depleted, but food preparation is very important to increase absorption in a tired and inflamed body. Animal meats that are high in gelatin, such as short ribs or oxtail, require a longer cooking time, but they are easier to digest than muscle meats like steak, which can sit in the stomach like a rock.

Pasture-raised animals are exposed to much more sunlight, which plays an important role in vitamins D and K2 production. While growth hormones are used to fatten up animals in commercial farming, these are not used in pasture-fed animals; however, some well-known grocery stores get their meat from farmers who "finish off" their cows with three to six weeks of corn. Check with your butcher or farmer to see if corn feed is in the meat you purchase, especially if you have neurological Lyme-associated symptoms (such as seizures, spasticity, facial palsy, or nervous ticks). Corn can make neurological symptoms worse.

THE CONUNDRUM OF RAW DAIRY

Dairy can be very problematic for those who are dealing with chronic Lyme and mold-related illnesses, and it is best avoided or restricted. Some individuals, especially of European descent, tolerate home-fermented, raw milk products (kefir, for example) that are exceptionally nutrient dense, support a needed diverse gut flora, and provide bioavailable vitamins and healthy fats.

If dairy is tolerated, it is best to only choose goat or sheep sources because their casein content is much lower than that of cows.

Dairy increases mucous production, and worsens neurological and cognitive symptoms (including having a morphine-like effect on the brain, resulting in brain fog). Dairy, with its naturally occurring sugar lactose, also feeds chronic sinusitis, vaginal yeast, or ear infection and worsens constipation or other gut issues. Dairy products, excluding butter and eggs, can escalate Lyme-related, digestive, neurological, and respiratory symptoms.

After prolonged antibiotic use, lactose intolerance is common. It can be inherited or acquired, especially with early disruption of the gut flora. It is a good idea to do a self test by eliminating all dairy products to see if you experience improvements in your health. If you do, you know that dairy is a problem for you and is best avoided at this time.

If dairy is not tolerated, coconut milk or coconut kefir might be an option. Full-fat coconut milk (Native Forest brand is organic and packaged in a BPA-free can) can be combined with dairy-free kefir (Inner-Eco brand) to create your own homemade dairy-free kefir or yogurt. Again, just because it is a dairy-free option does not mean it is the ideal option for you.

With all new food substitution introductions, start with a small dose first and check your heart rate. If your pulse rate increases suddenly or you notice flushing in your face and ears, then that food choice is not a good one for you at this time. You could also dab some prepared food on the sensitive skin on the inside of the wrist to see if there is a skin reaction. The body does not lie; if it does not like a food, it will react. Also, check your face in the mirror: If you notice flushing, redness, and warmth in the face and ears after eating or drinking something; this indicates an increase in histamine, which can be a problem for many individuals. The body does not lie.

BIOAVAILABLE PROTEIN: HOMEMADE BROTH AND STOCK

Nutrients in meat, poultry, or fish broth are easy to absorb, and they assist in healing a leaky gut and stabilizing blood sugar. These are staple foods in therapeutic gut-healing diets, such as the GAPS Diet, the Specific Carbohydrate Diet, and the Low FODMAP Diet.

Broth is a general term that describes a soup made with marrow bones (my favorite), meat, pig's feet, or chicken feet, or different types of bones. Traditional bone broth is made from various types of bones, and it can be cooked for up to two days.

If you find you get headaches from the broth or have a glutamate or histamine intolerance, chicken meat or fish broth might be a better option. Meat stock made with whole chunks of beef or chicken is also a great base for vegetable soups or stew. This type of broth is often better tolerated if broth from cartilage does not agree with you. Cooking times are shorter for vegetables, poultry, and fish than for lamb or beef bones. When living with Lyme, meat broth or marrow bone broth with shorter cooking times (four to five hours only) is better tolerated.

From my professional experience, I see very good results in clients who add broth from various sources to their daily diet. It has nourishing properties, offering a delicious, nutrient-dense, and bioavailable protein source. A cup of chicken, turkey, or meat broth is easy for a compromised gut to digest and absorb, even during a herx. Homemade broth is always best; store-bought broth can be too high in sodium and may include spices that irritate your immune system.

With long-term antibiotic use, gut health can be fortified by drinking two to three cups of broth daily. Add a few leaves of Atlantic-sourced seaweed into the broth while cooking; the iodine will make the thyroid happy, will increase too low blood pressure, and will provide needed trace minerals for the body. (Avoid adding seaweed if diagnosed with Hashimoto's thyroiditis—even though the thyroid needs it—or if a known iodine sensitivity exists.)

When I cook my bone broth, I take a big pot and fill it with two pounds of marrow bones and add water so that the bones are well covered. Then I add some sea salt, bay leaves or seaweed leaves, and three tablespoons of raw apple cider vinegar. After it has come to a boil, I turn the stovetop down to a simmer for the next few hours. While it's cooking, I skim off the brown foam that forms on top of the liquid and toss it away.

I sometimes vary the recipe by adding herbs, and then I fine-tune it with spices or sea salt once I have carefully drained the liquid from the bones into a porcelain container. I do not cook bones beyond four hours, because I am prone to headaches when exposed to excessively high amounts of glutamate (or hydrolyzed protein in collagen, or gelatin powder supplements).

The gelatin and bone marrow from the bones from free-range animals are extremely nutrient dense, with vitamins, healthy fat, and minerals, and they help heal a leaky gut. The bone marrow in the core of the bones is an important part of the immune system, and it will help our immune system. Keep in mind that bone marrow is extremely rich in saturated fat that cannot be tolerated by many people whose liver and gallbladder are challenged.

Once the broth has cooled down in the porcelain container, the fat solidifies into a white layer on top. You can scrape off the fat, and the bone broth will not be as rich anymore; that might be best for you at the present time. Depending on your tolerance, choose how you can best digest the broth, in the full-fat or lower-fat version. Try different bone choices, including neck or tail bones, fish bones or heads, or even pig or chicken feet, which are great sources of gelatin.

Bone broth is a terrific, nourishing, whole food option that can be frozen. It is very versatile to cook with, or you can simply enjoy it in a mug. Farmers' markets sometimes sell stock or broth, but it is best to use homemade broth so you know exactly what is in your bowl or cup, especially if you have many sensitivities.

Benefits Of Broth, Meat Stock, and Bone Broth

- Easy to digest and to absorb
- Heals a leaky gut
- Great source of calcium, magnesium, silica, and trace minerals
- Great source of collagen and glycine (for glutathione production)
- Supports blood sugar balance (add vegetables)
- Great for joint and tissue repair
- Helps maintain muscle tissue

Regarding monosodium glutamate, MSG, and bone broth: It is important to note that glutamic acid is a natural by-product of the breakdown of protein in bone broth cooked for many hours. This is why I restrict the cooking time of bones to a few hours, depending on whether I use, for example, chicken bones or marrow bones.

With any neurological, nervous system, or behavioral challenge, a sensitivity to excess glutamate must be considered. Too much accumulated glutamic acid has a neurotoxic impact on the brain, making Lyme-associated symptoms worse. It can manifest in seizures, anxiety, migraines, vision disturbances, and insomnia.[3] If this resonates with you, broth from meats is a better option than bone broth.

ORGAN MEATS: PASTURE-RAISED ONLY

Organ meats are super foods rich in cholesterol, minerals, and vitamins, especially vitamin A, B12, D, E, copper, and iron. If your hemoglobin is low or you have excessive bleeding with your menstruation or blood loss with gastric inflammation, organ meats are whole food options to support your blood building ability, iron levels, and energy. But when living with Lyme, these rich foods might not be an optimal food option for you, or you might only tolerate very small amounts.

Pasture-raised animal liver contains the essential fatty acid DHA and cholesterol, which are very nourishing for cognition, neurological function, and decreasing brain inflammation. Vitamin A is in a bioavailable form, which supports eye health and boosts and supports the immune system.

I am aware that organ meats are not a favorite food for many, and they cannot be digested by those with a challenged gallbladder and liver function, but consider that a weakened digestion can limit your tolerance for foods that support good health. Ox bile salts facilitate the breakdown of fatty acids, and there are also lipase enzymes that are found in quality digestive enzyme supplements.

FREE-RANGE EGGS AND POULTRY

Antibiotics, toxins, and growth hormones in commercial poultry and its by-products irritate and stress the challenged immune system, gut flora, and liver. It is best to avoid all commercial poultry. Unhealthy, factory-raised chickens or turkeys will not support our health; instead, they contribute to inflammation, hormonal imbalances connected with estrogen, and toxicity in the body. The hormonal implications affect adults and children, and the estrogenic growth hormones contribute to increased breast tissue in boys and breast cancers in men.

Chickens should be running around freely, picking up worms, little stones, bugs, and other organisms in the pasture. Chickens have varying colors and the hardness of their eggshells vary. If they are fertilized, even better; the egg yolk will be a bright, rich yellow or orange. Duck eggs can be a great alternative, but they are more difficult to find in stores.

If you tolerate eggs, it is best to purchase only free-range poultry and pasture-raised eggs from the market or a local farmer. Egg yolks are a great source of bioavailable vitamins and choline, which is very helpful when dealing with any chronic ailment, digestive trouble, or mood disorder. (I like to add raw egg yolks to protein shakes.) The egg white is a great source of sulfur that is needed for detox, production of glutathione, and elimination of heavy metals.

If you are sensitive to eggs, do a self-test and see if the egg white or the yolk (or both) give you trouble. Sometimes the yolk can be tolerated, but not the egg white. Commercial eggs can include more food sensitivity triggers because GMO corn and soy (and who knows what else) are in the chicken feed. It may be these factors, not the actual egg proteins, that are triggering an immune response.

When it comes to the whole bird, choose only free-range chicken or turkey. Do check into the feed, as farmers might use soy and corn in the feed during winter months. Duck is another option; however, it can be too rich for some. A little duck fat might be tolerated as a healthy fat alternative in a homemade meal.

Chicken fat has antimicrobial properties, and many of my Lyme patients have had no digestive trouble with homemade chicken or turkey stock. Prepare the meat, boiling or roasting the chicken, and then use the leftover bones and skin for a homemade chicken broth. That will help heal the gut too, and it is a bioavailable protein source. (Be sure to add sea salt.)

When preparing poultry, remember that not everyone can tolerate certain herbs or spices, so go slow and see what you can reasonably consume. If you tolerate fresh garlic and onions, add them into your soup as well; both have anti-microbial and anti-Lyme properties, and they support your detox and circulation. Other medicinal, antimicrobial herbs and spices that can add a nice taste to your broth are rosemary, thyme, turmeric, cayenne, oregano, sage, fenugreek, fennel, savory, basil, and black pepper. Fresh-cut herbs are less potent than dried herbs, and turmeric is best absorbed in the presence of black pepper. But, some individuals do not tolerate turmeric, hot spices, or black pepper.

NUTRITION FROM THE OCEANS

Wild-sourced and coldwater fish are the best options for seafood. Frozen or fresh fish from the ocean is best, especially herring, wild salmon, and mackerel, which are loaded with healthy fats. Mercury is a concern when consuming wild fish, so it is best to choose smaller fish, such as sardines. (Other options are to include parsley or cilantro with the meal, or to supplement with spirulina or chlorella.) If you are on a tight budget, or just for convenience, consider consuming canned wild salmon, anchovies, or sardines (in BPA-free cans). Sadly, our oceans and rivers are polluted with toxins, heavy metals, prescription drugs, plastics, waste water, sewage, and runoff from commercial agriculture and industry. Traces of these ultimately end up in our body.

Shellfish is mostly farmed and fed with contaminated food pellets, and with a compromised gut and liver, it is a high-risk food for many. If you are living in coldwater areas, such as Maine or the Canadian coast, you will have better access to wild shellfish. Many with chronic Lyme do not tolerate shellfish because it can be tough on the liver, so it is a caution food. Accidental food poisoning is also possible, so use caution if you eat shellfish and consider increasing probiotics after a meal.

As a health consultant, I would advise against eating raw fish. A healthy body can eliminate harmful pathogens that come into our bodies with food, but a compromised immune system in the gut cannot. With a compromised gut from antibiotic use, indigestion, or Lyme symptoms, you are much more susceptible to picking up harmful bacteria and parasites in foods. Our stomach acid is the first line of defense; if you are taking any acid-blocking medications or have digestive troubles, this opens the door for food-borne pathogens to proliferate, creating symptoms that are not directly related to the Lyme infection. If you do eat sushi, make sure to take some probiotics just in case you picked up some harmful microbes.

Do your best to avoid farmed fish that is laden with hormones, antibiotics, colors, preservatives, and other sources of additives and pollution. Also, avoid all processed seafood (or other foods) containing soy or vegetable oils, "natural flavors," hydrolyzed protein, or citric acid. Check the labels: These ingredients are toxic, hormonal disruptors, they contain MSG, and they stress the liver and brain, causing indigestion, burping, and headaches. With chronic Lyme, it is safest and healthiest to prepare foods *at home.*

WHAT ABOUT SOY?

In traditional diets, fermented soy was eaten as a condiment, not as a protein replacement. It is a bioavailable source of protein, phytoestrogens, and vitamin K2. The fermentation process neutralizes plant toxins that are thyroid inhibitors. Soy, in traditional diets, was mostly eaten in small doses and in conjunction with seaweed, its minerals providing thyroid support. Fermented organic soy is acceptable in the forms of miso, natto, and tempeh; however, most of my Lyme patients are sensitive to foods and supplements that contain soy.

Popular unfermented soy foods will block absorption of zinc, calcium, magnesium, and B12—all of which are often already deficient when dealing with Lyme-related infections. Soy protein and soybean oil is prevalent and hidden in many commercial and organic foods, contributing to increased sensitivities.

Soy, with its natural estrogenic properties, is controversial. The debate continues, especially as soy formula, in soy protein isolate form, is consumed by twenty to twenty-five percent of infants in the US.[4] This raises the potential for hormonal and thyroid disruption, reproductive consequences, early onset puberty, and sexual dysmorphia, which are associated with excess estrogenic exposures during formative years. Estrogen dominance is of great concern today for all children, men, and women because it is implicated in weight gain, diabetes, obesity, PMS, fibroids, and cancers, to name a few. Yet it is essential to discern between naturally occurring phytoestrogenic properties in traditional foods, such as edamame or miso, compared to the chemical estrogens in plastics, pesticides, and processed foods.

I generally do not recommend soy for my clients because of its underlying endocrine, nutrient, and thyroid-disrupting properties (unless it is part of their traditional ancestral diet and consumed in limited amounts). If you do tolerate and enjoy fermented soy, add some sea vegetables, such as seaweed, into your miso soup to help the thyroid (unless you have Hashimoto's). Natto and tempeh are also acceptable fermented sources. Keep in mind that soy is one of the top five food allergens and many with Lyme have no tolerance of foods or supplements that contain soy.

Simplify Protein: The Top Three Takeaways

1   Quality matters: Choose pasture-raised meat, poultry, and wild fish.
2   Integrate broth, stock, and eggs yolks into your nutritional arsenal.
3   With each meal or snack, include a protein source.

Lipids: Fats and Oils

There are many great nutrition books on the market explaining the different fats and oils, or *lipids*, yet when living with persistent Lyme, there are certain factors to keep in mind. Some individuals cannot tolerate fats and oils, and this can be connected to a Lyme-associated infection. In addition, gallstones, medical treatments, birth control pills, and nonalcoholic fatty liver syndrome can also affect the ability to digest fats.

If you are going through a tough cycle in your Lyme, with severe nausea and possibly diarrhea, avoiding fat is a temporary therapeutic measure. In some cases, a low-fat diet is advocated because of a specific Lyme-related infection; however, fats and oils are essential for health.

They enable the function of the nervous system, hormones, digestive system, and physical structure. In our body, healthy fats and oils are used as a transportation vehicle in the bloodstream, shuttling vitamins, hormones, and minerals in and out of our cells. The brain needs fats to function well and for nerve protection against toxins and infections. How well we support our body with a variety of healthy fats and oils will have great bearing on how we deal with Lyme-related infections, which invade and harm our cells.

Bile salts, which are made from cholesterol in the liver, are needed to emulsify all fats in the diet. The addition of ox bile salts, probiotics, phosphatidylcholine, and specific digestive enzymes can ease symptoms related to challenged fatty acid digestion. Common symptoms include bloating, back pain, stomach pain, belching, gas, or diarrhea. It is through bile that toxins, dead debris from infections, metabolized meds, and pesticides are eliminated from the body. Any ox bile supplementation must be done under the supervision of a qualified practitioner.

Healthy fats from plant and seed sources, such as organic cold-pressed olive oil, macadamia oil, avocado oil, and unrefined palm oil, are often easier to metabolize for those with compromised digestion or with nausea related to Lyme infections and antibiotic treatment. Plant oils can be incorporated during food preparation and cooking, or they can be carefully poured over steamed vegetables on your plate. When cooking, only use these oils over low heat. Oils oxidize at higher temperatures and lose their health benefits. Oxidized oils create more inflammation in the body.

Healthy fats from animals, fish, poultry, nuts, seeds, and plant sources are essential to induce satiety, brain health, and blood sugar balance. They do not make us fat, and they do not clog up our arteries, but processed foods with partially hydrogenated vegetable oils, excessive refined starches, and sugars do.

Fats are required for the optimal absorption of vitamins A, D, E, and K and can be found in bioavailable form in animal, venison, and poultry. Fat-soluble vitamins are needed to aid microcirculation to the eyes, kidneys, and heart and play an important role in hormone and bone production. They also support healthy immune function, and we need as much immune support as possible when dealing with Lyme disease and a suppressed immune system. Free-range animals have the optimal ratio of anti-inflammatory omega-3 fats to omega-6 fats.

Some individuals do better with heavier fats from animal foods, while others require lighter fats and plant oils. For some, healthy fats can also include fermented dairy products such as kefir or goat yogurt, others prefer palm oil or coconut oil. (To fully customize my client's nutritional pathway, I utilize the Healthexcel System of Metabolic Typing; dietary modifications must be made according to present tolerance.)

Lipids include fats, phospholipids, and steroids, and they do not dissolve in water. (Wax is also a lipid, and examples include leaves of plants, bees wax, or the wax in our ears.) In our body, cholesterol and phospholipids, such as inositol, phosphotidylcholine, or phosphotidylserine, all play an important role in energy storage, sex hormones, steroid production, and maintenance of cell membranes. Fats from our daily diet are divided into saturated and unsaturated fats, and they are needed to dissolve and store vitamins A, D, E, and K. As you can see, our body requires a variety of fats and oils to support its various needs.

Healthy membranes should be shiny and glisten like rain drops and not be sticky with ragged edges. Phospholipids are important structural components for cell membranes. They create a protective barrier for the cell, but they also allow cells to be flexible. Without these, our cells would collapse. Imagine that membranes are like bubbles and can take on different shapes without popping. If membranes get damaged or pop, the cells die.

If there is a lack of essential fatty acids in the diet, membranes become weak and porous. Infections, toxins, and chemicals can easily penetrate weakened cell membranes and gain entry into the cells. There, they can create dysfunction at DNA level while also damaging its multiple structures, including its energy sources, called the *mitochondria*. This is associated with chronic fatigue. It is important to note that antibiotics and inflammation damage the mitochondria.

The Standard American Diet, with prevalent use of commercial vegetable oils, contains a high amount of heat-damaged omega-6 fatty acids in comparison to omega-3 fatty acids. This ratio makes blood platelets stickier, lowers HDL cholesterol, increases inflammation in the blood vessels, raises blood sugars, and will harm the brain, gallbladder, and liver.

All excessive heat used in pasteurizing, deep-frying, and use of a microwave damages the membranes of foods—just like it damages your cell membranes. This creates excessive oxidation in the body and is a key factor of aging. Too much oxidation creates health problems, just like a fire that burns out of control. Membranes become leaky, misshapen, and they lose their protective ability against infections. Think of membranes as being part of your immune system.

Man-made fats and partially hydrogenated vegetable oils are not healthy— they clog up the arteries and make membranes rigid and stiff. Nutrients cannot get in, toxins cannot get out, and the cells cannot communicate with each either very well. Man-made fats include cheap vegetable oils in clear plastic bottles that have been heat-treated and chemically altered to prevent rancidity and to facilitate a very long shelf life. They stay in our body for a long time. I would avoid all canola oil because it is processed rapeseed oil that has undergone treatment with a toxic hexane solvent, sodium hydroxide, bleach, and natural waxes.

A diet high in trans fats can lead to heart disease, insulin resistance, and obesity. Trans fats are hidden in many popular foods, including peanut butters, crackers, granola, and snack bars. They allow premature aging of cells on the outside and inside of your body.

Margarines, spreads, butter substitutes, and heat-treated vegetable oils contain long-chain fatty acids, which cause cell injury. These long-chain fatty acids become part of a structure called *lipid rafts* that are functionally important for harmful agents. In addition, *B. burgdorferi*, or Lyme disease, can siphon cholesterol from cells in the body to support their existence and, thus, persistence.[5] Viruses also use lipid rafts as a mode of transportation through porous membranes where they wreak havoc at DNA level. This is studied in diseases such as ALS, Parkinson's, and Alzheimer's.[6]

SATURATED FATS: HEALTHY FATS

Saturated fats, though vilified in commercial medicine and in the media for the last fifty years, are nutrient-dense foods. These fats are solid at room temperature and more stable in the presence of heat. Egg yolks, lard, duck fat, butter, tallow, ghee, coconut oil, MCT oil, palm kernel oil, and palm oil are all healthy fats. They all provide a wealth of nutrients, yet sadly many still believe that these fats cause heart disease and strokes. They not do not.[7]

Saturated Fats from Animal Products

Butter is a great source of butyrate, short-chain fatty acids that chop through harmful long-chain fatty acids, maintain gut barrier integrity and provide an energy source in the brain (ketones). In addition, it is a great source of bioavailable vitamins A, D, and K2. Organic, especially raw, butter is a health food.

Egg yolks are a great source of choline (and vitamins A, D, and B12). Choline is a component of phosphatidylcholine, which is an integral part of the cell membranes. Choline is also part of acetylcholine, affecting brain function, mood, and memory. All this health-supporting nutrition is contained in animal-sourced foods with saturated fats and cholesterol.

Saturated fats from animal sources are preferred nutrition for the heart and brain. Over half the brain is saturated fat, and it needs this type of fat to function well. Lamb, bison, venison, beef, and dairy by-products are all sources of saturated fat that include cholesterol and provide bioavailable vitamins A, D, and K2. With any developing brain, cognitive difficulties, brain inflammation, neurological illness, or disease, this nutritional consideration is important.

Plant-Based Saturated Fats

Coconut oil and palm oil are often well tolerated. Some people tolerate it in small amounts throughout the day. Coconut oil is easier than most other oils for the body to digest and absorb, without adding to liver stress. It contains lauric acid, which is antimicrobial, antifungal, and antiviral, so it supports the immune system as well as thyroid function. If you can tolerate coconut oil and coconut milk, add it into your daily diet; it will provide a healthy fat that supports your body and your brain.

Coconut butter, a puree of coconut flesh, can be a delicious option for many; however, some individuals are sensitive to coconut products. Coconut butter is rich in fiber compared to coconut oil, which is extracted from the flesh of the coconut and is very popular for supporting immunity. It is also an easy, readily available source of energy.

With its antimicrobial properties, coconut oil also makes a great toothpaste. By adding baking soda and organic peppermint oil, you can make a clean, toxin-free toothpaste at home. With thrush or other infections in the mouth, oil pulling with coconut oil is very helpful. Make sure to spit out the coconut oil (in the trash or outside, to avoid possible drain clogs) after you have swished and swirled it around in your mouth for ten minutes.

Cholesterol Truths—and a Few Myths, too . . .

Cholesterol helps the body repair itself. It is actually not considered a fat, but a steroid. It is a large, waxy, lipid-alcohol molecule that is very important for childhood development, health, and longevity. It is a vitally important building block for many processes in the body, including brain protection, bile formation, steroid hormone production, inflammation, and tissue healing. But cholesterol is not used for energy, unlike other fats.

It is a building material and carrier substance that shuttles nutrients to and from the liver into our cells. It is found only in animal-sourced foods and is produced inside the body.

There are two types of cholesterol. In the commercial paradigm, these are known as "good" and "bad" cholesterol; however, each one has an important function.

- HDL (high-density lipoprotein) moves cholesterol from the cells through the blood to the liver, where it is broken down.
- LDL (low-density lipoprotein) moves cholesterol from the liver through the blood stream to the cells.

Both types of cholesterol need a vehicle, and cholesterol uses a protein for its transportation in the blood. This protein is measured when you do a blood test with your doctor.

Cholesterol is needed for the formation of bile in the gallbladder, which is often already challenged by stress from the Lyme-related infections, birth control pills, medications, commercial foods, and toxins in our environment.

It is needed to make vitamin D in the presence of sunshine; however, as we get older, vitamin D production is not as efficient, especially with the use of excessive sunblock during summer months or the use of statin medications.

Our body produces cholesterol in the liver and in other organs, if it does not receive a sufficient amount from dietary sources. It is that important. Low cholesterol levels have been associated with increased risk of death with strokes, cancer, and other noncardiovascular illnesses.[8]

Some individuals have difficulty producing sufficient amounts of cholesterol, and certain Lyme-related infections will use cholesterol to create their own protective biofilms. If we eat cholesterol in foods, our body produces less; yet statin medications inhibit intrinsic cholesterol formation, affecting sex hormone production and mitochondrial function and increasing the risk of diabetes in postmenopausal women.[9]

Oxidized or damaged LDL cholesterol contributes to damage and inflammation in our blood vessels, especially in the heart and brain. With vector-borne infections, these might already be chronically inflamed. Additional damage occurs when we consume refined sugars prepared in the presence of heat, such as partial hydrogenation or pasteurization in processed foods, sugary heat-treated drinks, refined foods, and over-cooking of animal proteins by grilling, frying, searing, or roasting until they are crispy, with brown or black edges. This creates harmful free radicals, also known as *advanced glycation end products* (AGE).

In addition, toxins, heavy metals, and Lyme-related infections can become embedded in the tissues of the blood vessel walls, contributing to increased cardiovascular inflammation, congestive heart failure, atrial fibrillation, and plaque buildup. It is interesting to note that Lyme spiroketes can draw cholesterol from our own tissues for their own use.

Polyunsaturated Fats (PUFA: Omega-3-6-9, EPA, and DHA)

There are two main types of polyunsaturated fats (PUFA). These include omega-6 and omega-3 oils, and we need both in a ratio of four to one. It is important that one does not have too much of one and not enough of the other. These essential fatty acids are sensitive to heat, light, and oxygen. If exposed to any of these, the oils become oxidized; they contribute to inflammation in the body that can manifest in joint pain, weight gain, brain fog, and cardiovascular and other degenerative diseases. As these oils are heat sensitive, it is best to use more stable fats, including olive oil, butter, palm oil, and coconut oil for cooking purposes that involve heat.

Omega-3 essential fatty acids cannot be made by the body. They must be obtained from foods and are found in the fatty layers of coldwater fish, sardines, cod liver oil, fish oil, shellfish, krill oil, flaxseed oil, walnuts, and chia seeds. These anti-inflammatory, fatty acids support heart health, lower triglycerides, decrease the risk of strokes, and lower blood pressure. Omega-3 oils have blood thinning qualities and must be discontinued before surgery. A deficiency of omega-3 fatty acids can cause symptoms such as dry skin, joint pain, and irritability, especially with the excessive consumption of omega-6 fatty acids in the Western diet.

Fish oil supplementation is popular and is beneficial in lowering elevated levels of triglycerides.[10] Mercury and PCB contamination are a concern, but this must also be a concern with many other supplements. Essential fatty acids turn rancid quickly when exposed to air or light, so it is best to buy smaller bottles of a high-quality product and store it in a cool, dark place.

Long-chain omega-3 fatty acids called *eicosapentaenoic acid* (EPA) and *docosa-hexaenoic acid* (DHA) are essential for the wellness of the nervous system and the brain. EPA and DHA are anti-inflammatory essential fatty acids. These must not be confused with the harmful long-chain fatty acids from commercial foods.[11] DHA in cod liver oil is especially important for infants and children because their developing brains have a high need for these particular fatty acids. They are essential for anyone living with chronic Lyme, autism, learning challenges, and degenerative neurological diseases.

Alpha-linolenic acid (ALA) is a plant-based short-chain omega-3 fatty acid;

it is found in plant oils such as flaxseed, rapeseed, perilla, and walnut oil. The body uses ALA for energy, heavy metal chelation, organ regeneration, immune function, and free radical scavenging. (Excessive free radicals harm our cells and blood vessels.) The high content of lignans in flaxseeds also positively affects the estrogen metabolism in women.[12] They also have a profound impact on the testosterone (androgen) excess in PCOS in women and in prostate cancers in men.[13]

Gamma linolenic acid (GLA) is an essential plant-derived omega-6 fatty acid that plays an important role in membrane integrity, fertility hormones, skin and hair growth, bone health, diabetic neuropathy, and nervous system function. This fatty acid, too, cannot be made in the body, and it must be obtained from foods in our daily diet. Some good sources are evening primrose oil, black currant seed oil, sesame seed oil, and borage oil. Although it is a member of the omega-6 fatty acid family, GLA is metabolized differently than other omega-6 essential fatty acids and has anti-inflammatory effects.

It is important to keep in mind that we must balance the consumption of omega-3 and omega-6 oils, especially when living with chronic infections and elevated inflammation.

Monounsaturated fats are liquid at room temperature and semisolid or solid when refrigerated. These are the omega-9 essential fatty acids that are found in foods, but the body can produce these. Some of the monosaturated oils are olive, sunflower, safflower, and avocado oils. Nuts include almonds, macadamias, pecans, peanuts, and pistachios. Fruits include avocados and olives. Unrefined olive oil is a big favorite, and for good reason. Besides being around for centuries, it is a mainstay of the Mediterranean diet. It has tremendous healing properties for the inside and outside of the body. You can eat it and put it on your skin and hair, just like coconut oil. It supports heart health, increases HDL cholesterol, and supports membrane integrity and gallbladder function.

For cooking, it is better to use processed organic olive oil. Higher temperatures increase oxidation of the healthy heat-sensitive vitamins. The more pure the olive oil, the more oxidation occurs, which if consumed, can cause increased inflammation. Pour and enjoy organic, cold-pressed olive oil over steamed greens or salads. Avoid commercial corn, canola, soy, sunflower, and rice bran oils that have been partially hydrogenated and are toxic trans fats that clog up our arteries, brain, and cells.

Nut Butters and Plant and Seed Oils

Raw nut and seed butters are not exposed to heat and thus are less likely to be exposed to oxidation. These contain omega-3 and omega-6 essential fatty acids as well as gamma linolenic acid. Any heat processing can render the sensitive oils rancid, so it is best to keep them in the fridge. If you tolerate nut or seed butters, check the label—the fewer ingredients, the better. Quality organic brands include Once Again, Artisana, MaraNatha.

Nut and seed butters are a versatile resource of B and fat soluble E vitamins. They are low in sugar, they contain a variety of proteins and healthy fats, and they provide an array of healthy fat and protein options for snacks and meals. They make a great snack with a stick of celery, fresh apple slices, or rice crackers. If you do not tolerate nut butters, you might tolerate seed butters (e.g., pumpkin, sunflower, or sesame). Some individuals tolerate neither, especially if on a low-oxalate diet.

Brazil nut butters offer a great source of selenium, a mineral that is very important when it comes to Lyme-related infections, viral challenges, thyroid function, immune function, and detoxification.

Tahini, sesame seed butter, is one of my favorites. I use it in salad dressings with olive oil and raw apple cider vinegar or with lemon over chicken or fish dishes.

Sunflower seed butter is a great source of minerals such as magnesium, zinc, phosphorous, and copper, and it makes a satisfying addition to smoothies, salads, or a slice of sourdough or coconut flour bread. Make sure that no sweeteners are added, and I recommend avoiding any nut or seed butters sweetened with cane sugar or honey. Sprinkle on some sea salt instead.

Aflatoxins are poisonous fungi that affect nuts, seeds, and their oils. They have a particular affinity for peanuts; thus, I do not recommend consumption of peanuts, especially if mold and yeast concerns are already ongoing. I also urge caution with cashews. These too can provoke hives or other allergenic conditions. Storage of any nuts or seeds is a concern because of rancidity and mold exposures, which will feed any mold-related illness.

Storage of Healthy Oils and Fats

Quality matters: All oils should be fresh. A fancy bottle and higher price is not an indicator of better quality. A good oil induces a small tickle in the throat, or even a cough or two with its peppery or bitter polyphenols. Once opened and exposed to oxygen and light, oils start to become rancid. This is why it is better to buy a smaller bottle and replenish it frequently; rancidity increases inflammation. Many organic and cold-pressed oils do not undergo various heat and chemical treatments to increase their shelf life like harmful commercial vegetable oils. Also check that the oils are properly stored in the grocery or health-food stores. If not, do not buy it there, because it might already be rancid.

It is best to refrigerate certain nut and seed butters if the kitchen is on the warmer side. (Turn the jar upside down and then stir it a little while, mixing in the oil that settles on top.) These include borage oil, evening primrose oil, cod liver oil, fish oil, and flaxseed oil. Certain oils are more stable and do not require any refrigeration, but you should keep them in a cool place in your kitchen—away from the stove or a cabinet that gets a lot of direct sunlight. These include olive oil, ghee (clarified butter), sesame oil, coconut oil or butter, and palm kernel oil.

Simplify Fats: Top Three Take-Away Tips

1   Nourish yourself with a variety of unrefined fats and oils from the seed, nut, plant, animal, poultry, and fish kingdoms.
2   Consume cod liver oil for brain health at any age.
3   We need fats and oils to absorb vitamins A, D, E, and K.

How to Nourish Your Brain with Healthy Fats and Oils

With chronic Lyme, the brain and nervous system are severely impacted, resulting in multiple symptoms, including spasms, palsy, cognition challenges, memory loss, and multiple sclerosis- or autism-like symptoms. When you add the various exposures from gluten, sugars, secondary infections, vaccinations, and our excessive environmental pollutants to the condition, you can see that the protective brain membranes need long-term protection against recurrent daily insults. The brain is over sixty percent fat, so it makes sense that healthy fats are needed to protect the brain and nerves.

Grass-fed butter is a fantastic brain food. Its color should be a sunny yellow, reflecting the vibrancy and nutrition of the green grasses of the pasture (especially during spring).

Cod liver oil is a whole food source of bioavailable vitamin A and D. Both are important for immune function, bone health, and eye and brain function. It will assist in dialing down brain inflammation and improving cognition and brain function by providing DHA. Many individuals cannot convert beta-carotene (a precursor of vitamin A) into the ready-to-use form of vitamin A, thus cod liver oil is a great option. Remember to choose your product carefully; contaminated products are rampant. A great resource for information about cod liver oil is www.westonaprice.org. Remember that many oils make false claims regarding their ingredients and are contaminated with toxic materials.

Choline is very important for brain wellness. It plays a protective role for the membranes of the brain cells, and it facilitates absorption of magnesium. It is grouped with the B vitamins and is important for mood chemicals and muscle function. Choline is also important in pregnancy because of its role in facilitating membrane integrity in the form of phosphatidylcholine and because of its anti-inflammatory actions.

The brain can utilize coconut oil for energy. Thus, it is also recommended for neurological ailments such as multiple sclerosis, Lou Gehrig's disease, Parkinson's, and Alzheimer's. Insulin is not required for absorption, so coconut oil can provide a quick source of energy comparable to sugar, which requires insulin for the transport mechanism into the cell.

An energy-starved and inflamed brain is an unhappy, tired, and depressed brain. If insulin resistance or diabetes are also in play with Lyme-related infections, coconut oil is a helpful brain food. It can also be applied topically to the skin, hair, and nails. Coconut oil can be used in curries, over steamed vegetables, in a lentil salad, over quinoa, or in creamed buckwheat. Coconut milk can be used in soups, sauces, curries, shakes, and desserts. (Manufactured MCT oil, a medium-chain triglyceride oil from a blend of coconut and palm oils, is popular. It is helpful to increase energy, gut health, and cognition. However, it contains no or little lauric acid, which is a powerful whole food immune booster and brain energizer.)

The brain and nervous system need vitamins, too—but in certain ratios and with cofactors and enzymes that whole foods provide. B vitamins are very important for brain health and our nervous system, and they cannot be stored in the body; thus, we constantly have to replenish them. B vitamins are found in animal sources and plant sources; however, I recommend supplementation. With chronic stress, it is very likely that a deficiency is present. Choose a quality product, as cheaper supplements may use petroleum or coal tar as sourcing material. There are several whole food and nutraceutical options, but discuss this with your doctor, because certain genetic factors might require you to have higher therapeutic dosages initially.

. . . .

Wrapping Up

There are so many factors to consider. Take heart; if you eat from unprocessed whole food sources and carefully add oils and fats from a variety of animal, plant, nut, and seed sources, you will be on the right track.

Start slowly and carefully, with small quantities. Gradually increase oils and fats according to your tolerance, and, of course, according to what appeals to your palate. Each unprocessed oil and fat has a health benefit. Go slowly and listen to your body.

Digestion and absorption are key, and with Lyme plus coinfections and medications, this gets tricky. Depending on your infection and treatment, you might have to go on a lower fat diet; everyone is different.

Consider the actions tips below. Which one resonates with you?

Action Steps for a Healthy Diet

» Check off actions taken

☐ Eliminate all artificial sweeteners and simple and refined sugars from the diet (including fruit juices, soda, and alcohol).

☐ If you have been eating fat-free foods, integrate healthy fats and oils. This can include free-range butter, coconut oil, evening primrose oil (not if pregnant), whole egg omelets, avocados, nuts, nut butters, chia seeds, and palm oil.

☐ Check your vitamin D levels, both markers, in a blood test.

☐ Avoid all processed salt. Only use Himalayan, Celtic, or sea salt in your foods.

☐ Add a probiotic (and fiber supplement) to support your gut microbes that use fiber to create health-supporting butyrate.

☐ Hydrate well! Restrict coffee consumption to one cup per day (organic is best) to protect the adrenals.

☐ Herbal caffeine-free teas are a good alternative. Licorice, marshmallow root, ginger, cranberry, chamomile, and rooibos are options. Green tea is a healthy option.

We eat every day, multiple times a day. Food is foundational for everyone, no matter what. With your diet, you can lead the way to building resilience. But be patient with yourself and only make small, manageable changes along the way.

"Let food be thy medicine, thy medicine shall be thy food."

—HIPPOCRATES

Chapter Five

Energize—
The Blood Sugar, Food, and Stress Connection

If your blood sugar bottoms out, so do you. Blood sugar regulation is a roller coaster for many and greatly impacts quality of life. With energy dips and spikes during the day, you are "wired but tired," and hypoglycemic episodes can leave you feeling weak, jittery, and exhausted. You may have lingering fatigue during the day and then are wide awake at night and cannot fall asleep, despite being completely exhausted. Lack of sleep causes blood sugar problems, weight gain, as well as other symptoms. The all-too-familiar midafternoon slump can also affect your ability to concentrate on tasks. You can feel overwhelmed or pressured easily. The resilience and stamina reserves needed to go to battle daily are not available when you are experiencing blood sugar swings.

If you often wake up between 1:00 and 3:00 a.m., a common occurrence with hypoglycemia, it can be difficult to fall asleep again—especially if the mind is active with stressful thoughts or worries. Fevers and night sweats from *Babesia* can keep you up, or heart palpitations from *Bartonella* might kick in when you are trying to sleep. It is during these times, in the darkness of the night, that you can lose hope and wonder if you will ever get better. You might not be able to get to sleep until the early morning. No wonder you feel tired from the moment you get up in the morning.

You are not alone.

Cardiovascular, vagus nerve, and nervous system dysfunction can result in a faster resting heart rate and excessive low blood pressure upon standing. This is known as *POTS* (postural orthostatic tachycardia syndrome) and must be treated by a health professional. With this condition, you may also feel dizzy, cold, and exhausted. Hypoglycemia, dehydration, heavy metal toxicity, and nutrient deficiencies, such as a magnesium or vitamin B-complex deficiency, can exacerbate heart-related symptoms. Get yourself checked out by a cardiologist if you are experiencing any heart-related symptoms—a functionally minded and Lyme-literate cardiologist would be best.

Sugar cravings are not uncommon when stress is too high and an energy crisis is present. While the body is in stress mode, glucose (sugar) is the preferred source of energy because it can be converted quickly into energy. With ongoing stress, the body creates a new software program that runs on sugar because it needs quick energy, instead of using the more complex primal mechanism of burning fat as a fuel source. Glucose will provide a lot less total energy than fat, and the body will soon run out of energy and crave more sugar. By eating more sugar, you will crave more sugar. In comparison, the body fares better when fat can be used for energy, because it provides much longer-lasting energy without slumps or hypoglycemia.

Blood sugar balance is very much affected by what, how much, and when we eat. Besides too much sugar in the diet, hypoglycemia (low blood sugar) can also be related to dehydration, low mineral status, thyroid dysfunction, cortisol deficiencies, and medications.

To get a better understanding of how to manage blood sugar imbalances, it is also important to consider that blood sugar control is very much affected by how we respond, and adapt, to any perceived stress in our lives. Social stress, anxiety, unresolved emotional trauma from childhood or in adult life, work difficulties, family arguments, and other nervous system stimulants, including Wi-Fi, also adversely affect blood sugar balance.[1] It is important to see the big picture when living with persistent Lyme. Sleep matters greatly because a restless night can induce cravings for carbohydrates and a larger insulin response to starchy or sugary carbohydrates eaten in the morning. This promotes weight gain and increased inflammation.

Any perceived threat will induce the innate stress response that includes a rise in blood sugar as the body gears up in primal, protective survival mode. High blood sugar is followed by a spike in insulin that results in a dramatic blood sugar drop. Over time, chronic spikes and dips contribute to metabolic and hormonal problems. This is part of the complex picture of insulin resistance, weight gain, blood pressure problems, diabetes type 2, estrogen dominance, and leptin resistance. A common drug prescription for insulin resistance and PCOS is metformin, which depletes vitamin B12 and thus can contribute to neuropathy and memory problems.

Besides making dietary and lifestyle changes and practicing stress-reducing therapies, effective blood sugar support can include herbal supplements such as berberine (avoid with severe hypoglycemia), bitter melon, gymnema, and Korean red ginseng, all of which support kidney and liver function in addition to blood sugar balance and insulin sensitivity. (Korean white and black ginsengs are the same plant as the red ginseng; they are processed differently for different uses.) Minerals that are needed to regulate blood sugar and insulin include chromium, magnesium, copper, vanadium, manganese, and zinc, and these are deficient in our soils and foods today. Adrenal support is essential with all blood sugar concerns.

How To Use Nutrition To Balance Blood Sugar

- Avoid refined sugars, sodas, juices, sweets, syrups, and jams that contain genetically modified high fructose corn syrup (HFCS), an industrial food product. These are blood sugar spikers. HFCS is hidden under various names, including fructose and fructose syrup; however, it is a processed synthetic version, very different from naturally occurring fructose.
- Always include a source of protein and healthy fat when consuming starchy carbohydrates or fruit.
- Restrict daily fruit consumption.
- Aim for quality nutrition with regular meals, so your adrenals are not called upon to raise your blood sugar if you skip meals.

- Eat fiber-rich foods that start the conversion of carbs into sugar and prevent spikes.
- Integrate food eliminations to allow the gut to heal.
- Optimize nutrient absorption by chewing well; connect the brain with the gut.
- Support the brain and adrenal glands with whole food nutrition and healthy fats.
- Supplement with nutrients, herbals, homeopathic preparations, or healing arts to support blood sugar balance and adrenal function.

How Stress Impacts Blood Sugar Balance

The body requires physical and mental energy to withstand the stress associated with completing daily tasks, such as driving kids to their after-school activities, performing at work, taking care of family commitments, maintaining a complex supplement or medication schedule, planning and shopping for meals, preparing meals, and keeping house. We need energy, and food cannot provide enough nutrients to make adequate energy when you are dealing with Lyme- or mold-related infections.

Any viral, bacterial, or parasitic infection keeps the brain and body wired in a fight-or-flight stress response mode. While in this mode, the body is not concerned with digestion, reproduction, or detoxification. It becomes a labyrinth of dysfunction where different layers must be unraveled, and it takes time to implement changes.

Take a moment and reflect: Are you pushing yourself too hard in your daily activities? Do you have enough resting time? Do you rely on sugar, coffee, and maybe alcohol or smoking, which initially make you feel wired with fake energy, but then you crash and feel even more tired? Do you feel guilty because you have lost interest in sex and feel you are neglecting your partner's needs? Are you spending too many hours with technological devices? These questions matter. When living with Lyme, excess stress siphons our metabolic and hormonal reserves, which prevents us from rebounding after infections and becoming well.

Our internal stress meter is primarily controlled by the pituitary and hypothalamus glands in the brain. The thyroid and ovaries or testes are also part of the stress hormone axis. All interconnect with the adrenal glands that sit on top of the kidneys. Think of this system like a tree trunk that begins at the top of your head and extends all the way down your trunk. These endocrine glands run the show and are closely linked with our blood sugar, moods, gut, and the immune system. They are greatly affected by persistent Lyme infections and mold exposures.

When our brain perceives stress of any kind, the nervous, immune, and endocrine systems jump into fight-or-flight survival mode. This primal response, which is initiated by the reptilian brain in the basal ganglia, can be triggered by a spirochete infection, low blood sugar, a stressful thought, trauma, exposure to EMF, or an injury. The perceived stress triggers a complex chain of events: The hypothalamus calls the pituitary and adrenal glands into action. Adrenaline is released from the adrenal glands. It increases the heart rate, enabling the heart to pump more oxygen to the muscles. Blood pressure increases, concentration sharpens, and our blood sugar increases so that we have energy available to physically escape the perceived threat. However, in most cases, there is no physical threat. Without physical activity, our blood sugar stays elevated; this is also known as *hyperglycemia*.

High blood sugar is poison to the brain. In response, the brain instructs the pancreas to release insulin to lower blood sugar. Insulin, a fast-acting hormone, moves sugar out of the blood stream and into our cells where it can be used for energy. When the level of glucose in the blood has decreased appropriately, production of insulin stops. The body has its innate checks and balances. But if the cells are already full of sugar, the cells ignore insulin's signals. Now the pancreas will keep pumping out more insulin, and insulin levels in the blood rise. This hyperinsulemia is not a good situation either, as elevated insulin levels in the blood are harmful too, and the pancreas gets stressed. Excess insulin is inflammatory, promotes cardiovascular risks and cancers, type 2 diabetes, PCOS, feminization of men, damage to the mitochondria, and storage of body fat, and makes it difficult for our body to burn fats for energy. With prolonged stress from vector-borne infections, multiple metabolic processes go awry, inflammation goes up, and our energy goes down.

Additional stress from other sources directly influences our ability to become well. These can include—

- The foods we eat, such as sugars, starches, processed foods with pesticides, and rancid fats
- How we eat during the day (skipping meals versus nourishing on a regular schedule)
- Lifestyle factors, such as sleeping habits, lack of movement, and smoking
- Mind-body issues (i.e., the emotional, spiritual, and mental stress we experience in our daily lives affects our bodies)
- Financial stress
- Job performance (inability to work)
- Relationships at home and at work
- Medications, including antibiotics, steroids, and the antianxiety and other drugs for insomnia
- Emotional, physiological, and family relationship stress
- Secondary gut infections and fungal infections
- Heavy metal toxicity
- Food intolerances, a leaky gut, and compromised gut flora
- Depression
- Anxiety

When it comes to stress and blood sugar balance, we must keep the whole person in mind, and with Lyme it becomes even more complicated.

Besides treating the underlying infections to lower the microbial load and to prevent flare-ups, add daily stress reduction in small, manageable steps. This can include taking a short break midafternoon, putting your feet up for a ten-minute rest, taking a bath with epsom salts before bed, making sure to eat breakfast in the morning, taking a probiotic with bifidobacteria, or eating organic vegetables. Even though the electromagnetic frequencies add additional stress, technology can be used to our advantage for health-tracking purposes. From a holistic perspective, there are numerous apps that can help in stress reduction techniques by providing biofeedback, heart rate, and sleeping rhythms. If you feel worse near electronics, avoid them as much as possible. Take small steps, but take them consistently; each one will help you.

Chronic Fatigue Busters: The Brain, Adrenal, Thyroid, and Mitochondria Connection

With chronic infections, the hypothalamus and pituitary gland in the brain can have altered function because of ongoing stress overload. Prolonged harmful exposures, including trauma, PTSD, and Lyme infections, all contribute to dys-regulation of moods and multiple brain mechanisms. Think of this like a switch-board that is experiencing short circuits and sparks when too many calls come in at the same time. Communication breaks down. Chronic fatigue, mood dis-orders, POTS (dysautonomia), and mysterious neurological pains often accom-pany this situation, and the individual is sometimes referred for psychiatric care. Yet in many cases an underlying vector-borne (e.g., *Bartonella*) infection is not considered. Often financial resources are a limiting factor for advanced testing.

The body is always trying its best, but with ongoing strain the brain down-shifts into a protective mode to conserve energy. When exhausted, the body and brain can only focus on basic survival mechanisms such as breathing or main-taining the body's blood pressure. As a protective measure, the brain instructs the adrenal glands to release less cortisol. The thyroid might also slow down to save energy, and the metabolism becomes sluggish. Now the body becomes burdened with toxins. The cells become too tired to function well, frequently causing sleep and mood disorders. The good news is that you can make multiple interventions along this complex path that will move you toward better health and increased energy, but it requires assistance and critical thinking from a Lyme-literate practitioner.

With persistent Lyme, the daily adrenal secretion of cortisol is often either deficient or excessive. The adrenal glands also produce our natural anti-inflam-matory and analgesic, cortisone. That, too, will be deficient with chronic stress. Sustained nervous system and hormonal stress is implicated in a myriad of dys-functions including—

- Hypoglycemia
- Weight gain and insulin resistance
- Gut dysbiosis
- Sex hormone imbalances, PMS, and menopausal symptoms
- Chronic inflammation
- Infertility
- Chronic pain
- Lyme disease with vector-borne infections
- Heavy metal toxicity
- Thyroid disorders
- Autoimmune challenges
- Chronic fatigue
- Mystery illnesses

Cortisol levels should be highest in the morning and decrease gradually during the day. Melatonin, produced in the pineal gland in the brain and the gut, should rise in the late afternoon. The melatonin and cortisol secretion pattern is often out of balance with persistent Lyme, and it contributes to ongoing sleeping challenges and fatigue. Elevated cortisol levels at night make it difficult to fall asleep, and low levels of cortisol in the morning make it a struggle to get out of bed. With suspected mold illness, testing of MSH (melanocyte-stimulating hormone) is advised.

Adrenal salivary and urinary testing is very helpful to assess current levels of cortisol, DHEA, and sex hormones that all are affected with chronic Lyme, creating secondary symptoms of ill health. Testing also provides baseline information regarding stress levels and adaptation, the Circadian rhythm, and blood sugar fluctuations. They are all interconnected in the landscape of Lyme.

Some consider the associated fatigue within the stress overload scenario adrenal fatigue; however, you can see that it is not only about the adrenals as it involves various glands, starting with the hypothalamus. For decades, we have used a model of adrenal saliva testing and an adrenal assessment of three stages of adaptation that included the alarm, resistant, and exhaustion phases. This is an outdated paradigm that is not supported by scientific evidence.

It is time to rename the concept of adrenal fatigue *HPA axis dysregulation,* which correlates with decreased resilience, lowered acute stress handling capacity, and disrupted cortisol patterns that are also implicated in neuropsychiatric hormonal imbalances, inflammatory illness, and sleep disorders. It is also high time that conventional medicine accepts this phenomenon and investigates root cause resolutions instead of relying on heavy-handed, long-term pharmaceutical therapies that come with addiction, side effects, and weight gain—and are often not effective in the longterm.[2]

Tired adrenals do not cause symptoms. Dysregulation happens in the brain, in the nervous system, in the tissues, with blood sugar balance, with sleep problems, with inflammation, and so on. This sophisticated perspective allows for better diagnostic and treatment options. Rather than stagnating with a reductionist viewpoint on adrenal fatigue, it is better to consider the scientific twenty-first century perspective: Low cortisol production is regulated and connected with the brain, not the adrenals. The adrenal response is complex; the downshifting of adrenal output is not regulated by the adrenals. Key components that affect cortisol output include—

• Ongoing stress, including infections, leaky gut, and food sensitivities
• Down regulation of the HPA axis
• Stimulants in the diet including sugar and caffeine
• Cortisol resistance in the body's tissues
• Steroid medications

Free form cortisol in the saliva is potent, but it gives an incomplete picture in regards to cortisol. Newer testing methods, such as the DUTCH test from Precision Analytical, test for urinary metabolites of cortisol, the active form, and cortisone, the less active form. We know now that salivary cortisol only makes up three to five percent of the body's total cortisol. It is possible to have low levels of free form cortisol in the saliva yet high cortisol metabolites in the urine, such as in insulin resistance, obesity, and chronic fatigue syndrome. This breakdown changes the way we perceive and support overall stress and adrenal function.

Any form of stress affects the kidneys and adrenal glands; they are closely related to all parts of the body, including the heart. Dehydration and constipation are the biggest challenges for kidney function. If toxins are not eliminated, they will keep recirculating, causing headaches, skin problems, hemorrhoids, weight gain, and inflammation. Spinal orthopedic pains are interconnected with challenged kidney or adrenal function; all back and knee joint pain (in conjunction with Lyme-related joint pain) must be seen in context with adrenal and kidney function. Hormone production, mineral and fluid balance, heart function, and blood cleansing are all connected to the adrenal-kidney complex known in Chinese medicine as the *kidney channel*. If you are experiencing water retention in your ankles, excessive urination, chronic pain, gut issues, and low blood pressure, you know your adrenals are challenged. It also affects the body's ability to mitigate inflammation and to get rid of heavy metals. With persistent Lyme, your adrenals are challenged.

Adrenal function plays an important role in our sex hormones as we age. In menopause, the adrenals are supposed to compensate for lowered estrogen and progesterone output from the ovaries. Tired adrenals cannot do that, and low sex hormones will contribute to mood disorders, sleep problems, weak bones, increased inflammation, and other symptoms that can be mistaken for Lyme symptoms.

Our adrenal glands need various nutrients, including vitamin C and B complex, besides cholesterol. In many cases, the diet does not provide sufficient amounts of vitamins and minerals, including organic copper. If you tend to bruise or bleed easily, this can be an indication that you are vitamin C deficient. Vitamin C also works closely with vitamins K and E, so you might be deficient in all three. Just like hormones, different vitamins work closely together in the body and taking a single high dose of one nutrient can upset a delicate balance. It is important to distinguish man-made and synthetic ascorbic acid from the naturally-occurring vitamin C complex that is required for adrenal function.

Ascorbic acid is only the preservative part of the whole vitamin C complex. Imagine it like the wrapper of a candy that prevents the breakdown of nutrients of the vitamin C complex. It has never grown in the soil and does not contain rutin, bioflavonoids, tyrosinase, and minerals of whole food complexes that create a functional vitamin C complex. Ascorbic acid is sold as a vitamin C supplement *but* is not a whole vitamin C complex, and thus it will not resolve a vitamin C deficiency in the body. Ascorbic acid will take nutrient reserves in your body to create a whole vitamin C complex, and that can induce further nutritional deficiencies. It is often produced from synthetic sources, including GMO corn or petroleum, so check the sourcing if you are supplementing. Whole food sources of vitamin C can include rosehips, citrus fruits, dark leafy greens, and select herbs such as parsley. In acute cases, especially when you feel a viral infection like the flu coming on, supplementation of ascorbic acid is helpful as an acidifier. However, too high a dose of supplementation can create loose bowels and affect oxalate production in the body.

Herbal formulations, flower essences, and homeopathic remedies are essential for adrenal support when living with Lyme. Glandulars are powerful supplements and can provide a jump start. Herbal adaptogens are terrific, especially with elevated or insufficient cortisol output; they have a modulating effect on the hormonal, nervous, mood, and immune systems, while also supporting daily stamina and mental clarity. Examples include ashwagandha, rehmannia, eleuthero (Siberian ginseng), and rhodiola.

Check in with a professional before using glandulars and herbs. Some are contraindicated with certain health conditions, autoimmune diseases, and especially with breastfeeding and pregnancy. Certain herbs are also contraindicated with sleep, heart, and psychiatric medications. Licorice root with glycyrrhizin is one of my adrenal, stress, and mood supporting favorites; however, it is contraindicated with high blood pressure. Combination herbal therapies and homeopathic remedies also have immune modulation and gut healing properties. With severe exhaustion, taking a short-term supply of whole adrenal gland concentrate (I recommend Desiccated Adrenal from Standard Process) will provide a helpful adrenal jump start.

The Thyroid Connection

The thyroid is the endocrine gland located just under your Adam's apple, the cartilage around your larynx. It is closely connected with our daily energy, as it controls the metabolism that affects our ability to get nutrients into the cells and harmful toxins out of them. It forms during the first trimester during pregnancy, so it is important that the mother's thyroid function is optimal before becoming pregnant. Thyroid hormones attach to receptors on the cell; this mechanism also occurs with other hormones, including insulin, estrogen, testosterone, progesterone, and cortisol.

No hormone in the body works on its own, and thyroid hormones work closely with insulin, cortisol, fertility, and other hormones. If you are ill, a hypothyroid or hyperthyroid condition can worsen your symptoms, especially with chronic Lyme infections that mask or imitate other health conditions. Too much or too little hormone secretion from the thyroid creates various symptoms in the body, affecting your heart rate and how well you feel, sleep, or think. It can also lead to hair loss, brittle nails, and dry skin. The thyroid affects our body temperature, enzyme function, digestive tract motility, and microcirculation to the eyes, kidneys, and heart; it even affects your moods. Incidentally, vector-borne infections prefer a cooler body temperature and thus can play a role in suppressing thyroid function, especially T3.

The thyroid is a cleansing filter for the body. It can be considered a detox gland as blood is continuously being filtered through it. However, heavy metals, viruses, and toxins can settle in the thyroid, affecting its function and hormonal output. Radiation also greatly affects the thyroid. Be sure to ask your dentist for a thyroid shield in case X-rays need to be taken. I also opt out of the security scans at the airport. Avoid radiation exposures when you can; they dial up the activity of infectious microbes.

It is important to consider that the thyroid might have already been challenged before you were infected with Lyme or coinfections. Perhaps you were already diagnosed with Hashimoto's or were already taking a thyroid hormone replacement. Be sure to monitor your thyroid function in optimal ranges, not lab reference ranges that are far too broad. But thyroid function is a clinical diagnosis, just like Lyme.

A sluggish thyroid can contribute to various issues, such as elimination challenges (slowed peristalsis), cold hands and feet, thinning hair, build up of low-density lipoprotein in the blood stream, and depression. Yet your labs are normal. An overactive thyroid can also create serious health challenges, including a faster heart rate, frequent bowel movements, insomnia, sudden weight loss, and restlessness.

Lyme microbes can attack various tissues in the body, including the thyroid. This can contribute to a hypothyroid condition that can develop into an autoimmune disease. In addition, gluten molecules in foods can travel through a leaky gut and settle on the thyroid gland. Infectious agents and food molecules can mimic our own cells. They confuse the immune system, which goes on the attack. This process is called *molecular mimicry*, and it contributes to dysregulation in which our own cells end up being damaged too. A well-known example is Hashimoto's thyroiditis, an autoimmune thyroid condition (or diabetes type 1 that affects the pancreas or ulcerative colitis in the colon).

Various hormones must be considered when assessing thyroid function. One of these hormones is the thyroid-stimulating hormone (TSH). This is not a thyroid hormone because it is produced by the pituitary gland after receiving a command from the hypothalamus. It is not a very reliable marker as it varies during the day and the pituitary does not rely on enzymes to activate hormones. TSH can be easily tested with a blood test. TSH signals the thyroid gland to secrete the hormone thyroxine (T4), the inactive form, which must be converted into triiodothyronine (T3), the active form. It is in this bioavailable form that the thyroid hormone is metabolically active in the cells. If T4 and T3 are too low, the pituitary, like a thermostat turning on, will release more TSH that stimulates the thyroid to produce more hormones.

Your levels of T4 might be optimal, yet the conversion to active T3 is insufficient because of a lack of enzymes and nutrients such as zinc, iodine, and selenium or a lack of vitamin E. In addition, elevated cortisol levels block the conversion from T4 to T3. (This is not considered in conventional endocrinology.)

Vector-borne infections affect thyroid function. Infectious microbes affect the conversion of T4 to T3. They prefer to operate in a cooler environment. . . .

The thyroid marker reverse T3, or rT3, is mostly produced in the liver. High levels (above thirty) indicate that the body is in stress mode, with elevated cortisol levels, and it is trying to conserve energy. Elevations in rT3 levels can also be an indirect marker of low stomach acid or selenium and low iron levels.

The thyroid is challenged by excessive toxic substances in the environment. These can include bromines in commercial baked goods; flame retardants in upholstery, mattresses, and furniture; medications, chlorine, chloramine, and fluoride in tap water; radiation from x-rays or TSA screening; and radioactive cesium isotope pollution from Japan's Fukushima reactor meltdown. Radiation lowers immune function and damages organs, glands, and mitochondria, altering DNA structure. The Endocrine Society has recently accepted the impact of environmental toxins on thyroid and hormonal function.[3]

Even if your thyroid labs are in optimal range, the following are clinical indicators that your thyroid is stressed:

- Foggy brain
- Depression
- A swollen tongue
- Yellowish discharge from nipples
- Brittle nails
- Constipation
- Low heart resting rate
- Fatigue
- A puffy face
- Feeling cold or cold extremities
- Hair loss
- Sleep problems
- Poor memory

Clinical findings matter greatly, just as they do in a Lyme diagnosis. You can also check your thyroid at home by doing the basal body temperature test at rest (Broda Barnes method) and cross-reference the result with your symptoms and lab findings.

It is not wise to treat thyroid challenges without also considering brain and adrenal function; they are all closely connected within our hormonal stress axis. It is important to understand that glandular fatigue is a *response to,* not the *cause of* chronic fatigue.

Check your thyroid function; have a blood test done with your physician. Make sure it includes all the thyroid hormones *and checks for the presence of thyroid antibodies.* Many doctors do not check the two antibody markers and miss that an autoimmune process is activated. Thyroid testing and reference ranges in commercial medicine are not preventative; instead, they allow for many individuals with a poorly functioning thyroid to fall through the cracks. With persistent Lyme, be vigilant about your thyroid function because it is a clinical stress meter in your body.

The Cellular Energizer and Immune Supporter: The Mitochondria

The mitochondria are implicated in chronic fatigue and cellular metabolism; however, their primary role is defense. Scientific evidence reveals that they are an important part of our innate and adaptive immune system, they control cell death if the cell is damaged, and they are located within cells as an antiviral and antibacterial agent. When threatened by foreign pathogens and toxins, the mitochondria induce an unfavorable environment to neutralize the harming pathogen or toxin in a protective process called *oxidation*. Their health and integrity directly affects our health and resilience involving a process call the *cell danger response*.[4]

Mitochondria convert carbohydrates, amino acids from proteins, and fats from our foods into glucose, which equals our energy. You might have heard about the Krebs cycle, electron transport chain, and adenosine triphosphate (ATP) production in biology class; well, it is in the many mitochondria that energy for all functions is produced.

A whole food diet that consists of many plants and healthy fats is essential to support this endogenous process. These provide nourishment with vitamins and minerals including zinc, selenium, magnesium, calcium, and other important trace minerals.

Consider the mitochondria are like tiny bacterial power plants. There are between 2,500 and 10,000 per cell, depending on what activity is required of the cell. Muscles that do a lot of physical work such as the heart and large skeletal muscles have a greater number of mitochondria, and this is why exercise is so important; with exercise, you increase the number of mitochondria in the cells.

We know environmental toxins, refined sugars, and herbicides in commercial foods pollute the membranes that surround the mitochondria and that Lyme infections, mold-related illnesses, and viruses severely impact and damage the

DNA in mitochondria. In addition, endotoxins released from infectious microbes called *lipopolysaccharides* are extremely poisonous to the mitochondria.

Antibiotics (bactericidal antibiotics), Tylenol, and psychiatric medications also damage the mitochondria. They affect their energy production and overall metabolic activity, which is also closely involved in the metabolism of vitamin D.[5] It is true that antibiotics can absolutely be life saving; there's no doubt about that. They certainly have their place in Lyme treatment, but not for all. Recent scientific findings on the implications of prolonged antibiotics treatment on the microbiome, mitochondrial dysfunction, overall effectiveness with persistent Lyme, and concerns with antibiotics resistance raise important questions about whether to continue this kind of drug treatment or not, and physicians are now more judicious in their use of it. Long-term antibiotic treatment is an individual's choice, and many do not tolerate its multiple side effects, including chronic fatigue.

Imagine if the workers (mitochondria) in the factories (your cells) are eating junk food, sitting all day, breathing toxic air, and working with harmful chemicals. The workers will be tired, get sick often, and underperform. They may even fall asleep on the job. No one is watching out for intruders or thieves. Without healthy mitochondria, no energy is produced. With damaged membranes, there is also no effective defense against toxins, chemicals, and infections that enter the mitochondria and the cell.

Many factors contribute to the silent inflammation that is associated with all degenerative diseases—Cell damage = inflammation = mitochondrial dysfunction = toxin accumulation cell death = chronic fatigue = disease states.

Contrary to popular belief, long-term supplementation with antioxidants interferes with the protective oxidation process within the mitochondria. Instead, the emphasis now is on phytonutrients in plants that stimulate or modulate immune function and targeted nutrients that enhance our DNA and detoxification pathways, and lower inflammation. Earlier I mentioned how we must protect our cell membranes with healthy fats and oils including choline in eggs, cod liver oil, and hempseed oil. This also matters for the two vulnerable mitochondrial membranes. In addition, anti-inflammatories in herbs or spices (including frankincense, green tea extract, resveratrol, and turmeric) dial down inflammation. CoQ10, D-ribose, Ala, zinc, B vitamins, and carnitine are helpful with increasing cellular energy, but please consult with a professional before supplementing.

. . . .

Wrapping Up

To make healing and recovery more doable, I have added action steps to give you realistic starting points. Chart your own roadmap according to your unique needs. Will progress be linear? No. Will you feel improvement over time? Yes. With chronic Lyme, there are so many different pieces of the intricate puzzle. I urge you to work with a knowledgeable health practitioner who fully understands the complex Lyme scenario, gut challenges, lymphatics, and drug interactions.

Choose a path that works for you, and only work with practitioners and doctors who listen to you and guide you in your decisions. You reap the consequences of your choices, so choose wisely. No one truly knows what you have been going through but you. Many will tell what you need to do, but listen to your inner voice of truth; that is your guiding light.

The body knows what to do, but it needs to be reminded of how to do it. It wants you to be well. Sometimes—especially after prolonged use of analgesics, antacids, steroids, and psychotropic medications—it can have forgotten what it should innately know. By improving organ and glandular function with whole foods, clean water, gentle movement, and rest, the body will start its own innate detox process. Emotional and social wellness comes into play as well, as any blockages in those areas can manifest as stress within the physical body.

Begin by taking action in one area where you feel that you can make changes without adding too much stress. It is important that you go slow and do not push yourself too hard. Remind the body that it is designed to heal by providing it with optimal nutrition, self-care, compassion, and love.

> "One of the biggest tragedies of human civilization is the
> precedents of chemical therapy over nutrition."
>
> —Dr. Royal Lee

Chapter Six

Action Steps to Support Your Blood Sugar Balance and Energy

1. Eat or Nourish Within the First Hour of Waking

Skipping breakfast creates a state of emergency in the body and creates energy slumps and blood sugar problems for the rest of the day. Not eating causes a yo-yo effect with your insulin and cortisol. You become more susceptible to sugar and carb cravings during the day, and you lose muscle. If you do not eat, the body will eat itself to compensate for a lack of nutrition.

Brain chemicals are made from amino acids, so it is easy to understand how a deficiency or an imbalance in brain chemicals can occur when proteins are redirected into energy production during a blood sugar crisis. This will affect your strength, resilience, energy, and moods. At rest, your brain needs about twenty-five percent of the glucose that is in your body to function. *Can you imagine how much more glucose it needs when it is stressed in an ongoing survival mode?*

By balancing your blood sugar within the first hour of waking, you are giving your body the energy it requires to accomplish daily tasks. We need nourishment for brainpower so we can maintain concentration and mental focus during the day.

The body requires us to eat or nourish soon after arising to ensure that optimal blood sugar regulation occurs from the beginning of the day, especially after a difficult night with restless sleep or pain. In many cases, there is an absence of appetite and a list of medications, supplements, or herbals that need to be taken on an empty stomach. If you do not have an appetite, a cup of broth with cooked vegetables, a room-temperature protein shake, or a cooked whole grain porridge with coconut oil (if tolerated) might be more palatable for you. If you tend to have a rough time in the mornings, you could prepare food the night before or make sure you have some leftovers or broth that you can heat up on the stovetop in the morning.

Foods that are rich in fiber optimize blood sugar balance, stamina, and nourish your gut ecology. Fiber slows down the absorption of sugar, preventing spikes associated with simple sugars that are abundant in processed foods, frozen foods, and fruit juices. Other choices include a protein shake with flaxseeds or chia seeds, a slice of gluten-free toast with butter and slices of turkey, unsweetened applesauce with sunflower seeds and coconut oil, or a cup of chicken broth with sea salt and cooked vegetable chunks. But keep in mind that for some, fiber can worsen underlying digestive ailments.

2. Include Protein, Healthy Oils, and Phytonutrients in Every Meal

Each time you nourish your body, keep it simple. You need a quality source of carbohydrates, protein, and fat with each meal and many different colors on your plate. It is better to have a variety of veggies than a large portion of one vegetable. If you have some chopped vegetables or fermented vegetables in a jar in the fridge, these make an easy addition (if you tolerate fermented foods). Dark leafy greens that are rich in chlorophyll and iron support blood building.

It is best to eat a few bites of protein first to stabilize blood sugars before eating starches or any higher glycemic vegetables on your plate. Make sure you chew well to stimulate gastric juices, digestive enzymes, and gallbladder activity. Every food group listed below is required by our body. Their interconnection helps us maintain a steady blood sugar while also providing us with energy during the day. Keep it simple:

- **Carbohydrates:** Simple or complex carbohydrate foods provide the glucose needed to raise low blood sugar, especially with tired adrenals and mitochondrial dysfunction. They provide the energy we need to break down protein and fat from food. We need carbohydrates in every meal, but not refined sugars. Restrict multicolored fruits and whole grains, which are caution foods for many, and choose seasonal vegetables.

- **Proteins:** We have a large variety of proteins to choose from. Proteins include pasture-raised animal sources that provide a good source of iron and B vitamins, their by-products, venison, free-range poultry, and wild-caught fish. Legumes, nuts, and seeds provide plant-based options. These contain the different amino acids that our body needs. Everyone is different and, of course, digestion ability must be considered. Proteins promote stable blood sugar and help curb food cravings.

- **Fats:** Fats and oils from animal, fish, plant, and seed sources (according to tolerance) foster the maintenance of blood sugar levels, add satiety, and can be burned for metabolic and brain energy. These are important to curb carb cravings. Just a note: peanuts and peanut butter are best avoided because they can be rancid or contaminated with mold spores.

3. Nourish With Small Portions Every Three Hours

To avoid blood sugar and energy slumps, it is best to nourish the body every few hours (about every three hours). It takes planning and practice, but you will feel better when you start to implement a regular eating schedule. A four-day food and energy diary is helpful for tracking your energy responses to meals and snacks, or lack thereof. Take note of energy slumps, carb cravings, mental concentration challenges, digestive troubles, or sleepiness after a meal. Your dietary choices and the time lapses between meals can play an important role in those symptoms.

With chronic fatigue you do not want to overwhelm the digestive tract with large meals that require a lot of energy to digest. It cannot handle large amounts of food at once, and you could feel even more tired if you overeat. Smaller portions at regular intervals will be easier for your digestive system to process. With compromised digestion and gastroparesis, initially, foods in liquid form are easier to digest. This can include a cup of pureed vegetables and chicken broth or a room-temperature protein shake with low-fiber vegetables and stevia. Chew the liquids to promote the pumping action that promotes drainage from the brain and secretion of enzymes in the digestive tract. It is a good idea to have some frozen soups on hand that you can heat up on the stovetop, especially if you are having a tough day.

Any hypoglycemic event causes severe stress on the brain and body, adding more strain to an already tired system. With ongoing fatigue and lower cortisol levels, eating on a regular schedule will go a long away to help manage blood sugar imbalances. In many cases, even just a few bites will raise and maintain blood sugar levels. In addition, the adrenals will not be called upon to raise blood sugar.

4. Plan Ahead

It does not matter if you are at home or traveling, planning ahead is key. When you are sick and tired, planning ahead takes more work, but it is worth it. Knowing that you have foods that are healthy and that meet your specific needs will ease mental stress; and it will enable you to manage your blood sugar, even when you are in an uncontrolled environment.

At home, stock your kitchen cabinets with healthy options such as organic beans, quinoa, coconut milk, healthy oils, sardines, wild salmon, and low-sodium chicken stock. With canned goods, seek out brands with a non-BPA lining. Keep frozen stock, soups, meats, and vegetables on hand that you enjoy. You never know when you might be having a rough day and can only handle a bowl of warmed soup.

When traveling, you want to have the foods, teas, and snacks that are right for you *with* you. You do not want to rely on a convenience store, hotel, airline, or airport to have healthy, allergen-free snacks—because they generally do not. When traveling by plane or train, you could pack canned wild fish, protein powder with stevia that you can stir into a glass of water, small sachets of organic almond butter, rice cakes, instant oatmeal, or whole food bars. If you are staying at a hotel, inquire about a refrigerator in your room so you can store your food safely.

If you travel by car, you can bring prepared foods with you and pack a cooler for the backseat. Add ice packs to the cooler and place your homemade foods in glass jars, or use a thermos for broth or soup. (Avoid cheap plastic containers with chemical estrogens.)

Because of security screenings at airports, bringing healthy options for snacks can be challenging when traveling by plane. And food at airports is certainly not health supporting. Pack healthy snacks in your work or travel bag. Being prepared will lower your stress and decrease food anxiety. Bring your own prepared foods such as boiled eggs; avocado chicken salad; rice or seed crackers spread with hummus or nut butter; grass-fed beef, turkey, or salmon jerky from Patagonia or Vital Choice; sliced vegetables or fruit in a Ziploc bag; coconut butter or almond butter packs; or a bag of seeds and nuts. These options will help you assist your blood sugar balance, even though you might get some questions from security personnel.

If you want to eat out, look for restaurants that offer gluten-free, free-range, and organic options. Investigate restaurants online or give them a call. Check out the menus online beforehand, and phone to inquire if they cater to food sensitivities such as gluten, dairy, corn, soy, eggs, and nuts; take note if they are responsive to all your questions. You want to know where you can eat safely when going out with family and friends or traveling.

Be very clear about your food sensitivities when ordering at restaurants or attending social functions. (You can always request steamed or grilled foods drizzled with olive oil to avoid harmful fats.) Always bring digestive enzymes with you, in case you are accidentally exposed to foods that you do not tolerate. If you have a nut or shellfish allergy, carry an EpiPen with you at all times—it can save your life.

5. Avoid Artificial Sweeteners, Alcohol, and Caffeine

Artificial sweeteners are neurotoxins. Think of neurotoxins as poisons that make your brain cells explode because they become overexcited and overstimulated.

Artificial sweeteners affect blood sugar balance and the insulin response, making your brain and body feel hungry.

When it comes to sweeteners, consider using stevia; however, keep in mind that it can break down biofilm and you could experience a herx. If you have ragweed, daisy, chrysanthemum, or marigold allergies, stevia is contraindicated (and also with blood pressure medications). Honey may have to be eliminated because it can feed fungal infections; yet local raw honey has enzymes, proteins, and nutrients that support skin healing and immunity, and a little may be well tolerated, especially Manuka honey. With any digestive ailment, stay clear of sweeteners with names that end in the letters *ol*, such as sorbitol or malitol; these can make your digestive symptoms worse. (However, xylitol is effective against biofilm and dental plaque in teeth.[1])

It is also best to avoid recreational alcohol consumption. Many with Lyme, postural orthostatic tachycardia syndrome (POTS), and digestive troubles have no tolerance for alcohol, even the alcohol in tinctures. Initially, alcohol is a stimulant, but it becomes a sedative that contributes to hypoglycemia, making you feel much worse after it is consumed. It is also a diuretic, and dehydration is a common concern when living with Lyme. Aldehyde, a chemical by-product in alcohol, contributes to palpitations, headaches, mood disorders, histamine symptoms, and brain fog. Alcohol also feeds fungal infections. It drains nutrient resources in an already compromised body, including B vitamins and minerals. Consumption compromises immune function, raises insulin, inflames the brain, induces hypoglycemia, and stresses the liver. Though some individuals tolerate alcohol, it is important to consider the accumulative side effects of recreational consumption. Alcohol increases systemic toxicity, nutrient depletion, and inflammation.

Stimulants like simple, refined sugars can deliver a great burst of energy and mental clarity that are soon followed by a crash. These substances rob the body of more nutrients and minerals, especially the B vitamins (in particular B6 and B12), magnesium, and zinc. Incidentally, many medications also siphon away these nutrients, and it is easy to understand how nutrient deficiencies creep into the nutritional landscape. A malnourished body and mind cannot become well.

With persistent infections, the body is very sensitive to all stimulants, especially if you have cardiovascular symptoms from infections. Caffeine will excite adrenal glands that are already challenged and can induce palpitations. With an irritated gut and reflux symptoms, coffee can create more indigestion or acidity, and it increases dehydration. If you have palpitations, severe blood sugar swings, or tend to feel jittery when drinking coffee, it is best to avoid caffeine.

If you enjoy your coffee and that cup is your "Zen moment," make sure it is a small cup and is not too strong, and drink it with a meal. Never drink coffee on an empty stomach, because it acts like a turbocharger on an already compromised system, and it can make you feel worse. However, organic coffee has antioxidants, and it can improve mental focus, muscular energy, and concentration. Adding coconut oil, medium-chain triglyceride oil, ghee, or grass-fed butter to organic coffee is helpful in curbing the cortisol and blood sugar response to caffeine.

Coffee interferes with sleep, even if you drink it in the morning. If you are doing cyclical Lyme-treatment and you already feel riled up, it is best to avoid coffee altogether. However, if it gives you a feel-good moment, enjoy a small cup with a meal before 12:00 p.m.

Caffeine-free herbal teas are a good alternative choice. They contain healing properties and antioxidants that encourage drainage, the nervous system, and good health. Licorice root teas will support adrenal and blood sugar function (avoid licorice if you have high blood pressure). Green tea is cancer protective and helps our heart health, but be aware that it contains caffeine, even if decaffeinated. With fungal issues or urinary tract problems, drinking of unsweetened cranberry, pau d'arco, nettle, or goldenseal tea can decrease uncomfortable symptoms; there are many other options beyond those, if these are not appealing. Marshmallow root, uva ursi, and slippery elm can be helpful with interstitial cystitis. Slippery elm, ginger, and peppermint ease gastric distress. Dandelion and milk thistle teas facilitate better liver function. My favorite loose-leaf teas come from Mountain Rose Herbs, but I also like to collect fresh leaves and brew them into a homemade tea. Gingko tea helps circulation and memory, and nettle leaves ease skin conditions. In addition, I also enjoy rooibos tea from my home country, South Africa. Choose what feels and tastes good for you; however, avoid iced teas.

6. Support The Mighty Mitochondria

A customized nutritional strategy and targeted supplementation is effective in increasing energy at the metabolic level by providing much needed vitamins, minerals, and fats to fuel the body, while also optimizing blood sugar levels. By lowering inflammation with healthy fats and decreased toxic exposures, we increase the function of our mitochondria in our cells.

Move to energize: Movement that incorporates mindful breath increases the number of our mitochondria, thus we create more energy when we move our bodies. It is certainly mood enhancing and can help with pain relief. Exercise of any kind also promotes the clearing of toxins by increasing the lymphatic flow, making you feel better. Implement a cautious conditioning program to reestablish bone mass and muscle strength for functional activities. Gentle daily movement can include a walk or breathing exercises while seated if you have a lot of joint pain, palpitations, and nausea or feel worse when your body temperature increases. If you are able to enjoy dancing and music, go ahead and join others at some fun social gatherings. Physical therapy can be helpful to build your strength with resistance training; however, use caution and monitor according to post-exercise fatigue. Mitochondrial renewal begins by moving your body on a daily basis; choose what resonates with you, especially when you are going through a tough time.

. . . .

Wrapping Up

Lyme and coinfections cause constant stress on the body and the brain, keeping you in a prolonged fight-or-flight response. Whole foods encourage healing and lower stress, and they contain nutrients in bioavailable forms that will not overwhelm the human body.

When living with chronic Lyme, it is prudent to investigate all health-supporting options, whether you choose a pharmaceutical approach or not. Supplementation is essential to support the body's various biological systems that are challenged by infections, medications, and antibiotics. With chronic illness, the body needs more nutrients than one can eat on a daily basis, especially since many nutrients are lacking in the soil and plants today.

But beware, certain supplements, such as a high dose of zinc, B6, or B12, can push certain mechanisms in the body into a faster gear, and if the body cannot handle it, it can result in a herx reaction. With ongoing fatigue, go slow and only add one supplement at a time to allow the body to adapt and respond.

Absorption is always a concern when taking supplements, and many have chemical fillers and inactive ingredients that prevent their absorption. Supplements in powder, liposomal formulation, spray, topical application, and liquid form are preferable for many. Be sure to consult with an integrative health professional before supplementing. You want to make sure they are not a contraindicated for medications you might be taking.

"Each patient carries his own doctor inside him. They come to us not knowing this truth. We are at our best when we give the doctor who resides within each patient a chance to go to work."

—ALBERT SCHWEITZER

Chapter Seven

Digest + Absorb = Nourish

All of my clients have digestive issues. If the gut is not well, we are not well. That is not surprising because our digestion, hormones, and immune and nervous systems are very closely connected. By the time a client consults with me, he or she has often already taken multiple courses of antibiotics, steroids, analgesics, antacids, and antifungal medications that have caused organ stress, nutrient deficiencies, and alterations in their ecological balance in the gut, sinuses, and urogenital tract. This allows troublesome opportunistic infections to gain a foothold.

What we eat and digest affects trillions of microbes in the gut. Eating healthy can shift the balance of power toward healing opportunities and better moods. This can manifest in a stronger voice, less pain, better sleep, or more energy. Restoring and maintaining the balance of power in the gut with more health-supporting microbes that counteract harmful microbes is key. This affects parasites, bacteria, viruses, and fungi, which keep each other in check. Eating nutrient-dense foods is a therapeutic intervention when living with persistent Lyme. Work on your digestion and your gut, and it will be able to work for you.

Our digestion plays an important role in our energy levels, yet we require a large amount of energy just to digest our food. A fatigued body equals fatigued digestion. The body needs easy-to-absorb nourishment, especially when it is in crisis mode. Broth and soups are a health-supporting part of a daily nutritional regimen when living with Lyme.

For many with chronic Lyme, digestive ailments were present before the initial Lyme-related infection; however, in others, gut problems started with the Lyme, *Babesia*, or *Bartonella* infection and long-term use of medications. Gut problems without appropriate dietary and flora-rebalancing interventions can morph into systemic ailments that mimic Lyme-related symptoms. Nervous system and psychiatric disorders, fibromyalgia, chronic fatigue, systemic toxicity, chemical sensitivities, allergies, autoimmune diseases, hormonal disruption, weight gain, insomnia, and sustained inflammation are all partnered with gut and digestive dysfunction, and all mimic Lyme disease symptoms. Remember, our gut affects every function in our body.

Lyme infections can directly infect the digestive tract. This can result in a Bell's palsy of the digestive tract with severe and debilitating consequences as nerves that govern transit are paralyzed. Infections such as *Borrelia*, *Bartonella*, and *Babesia* have an affinity for the gut, where they wreak havoc. Common digestive complaints include gastroparesis, reflux, abdominal pain, bloating, anemia, and intestinal blockages; these conditions can require a visit to the emergency room. The nervous system, digestive tract, gut flora, and gut lining are in need of therapeutic support, whether the individual is in active antibiotic treatment for Lyme infections or not.

The gut microbiome plays a major role in our ability to become well; since it houses over seventy percent of our immune system, it is largely responsible for our response to external infections. Our gut microbes produce vitamins that the body can absorb and use from the foods we eat. What we eat, the 100 trillion microbes in our body eat too—our food choices directly impact our gut ecology.

Our resilience and ability to thrive is very much dependent on the diversity of our gut microbiome, although the impact of the microbiome in illness, and wellness, is still not fully accepted in commercial medicine, psychiatrics, rheumatology, and pediatrics.

Prolonged drug and antibiotic interventions come with unwelcome side effects, which often remain problematic as they alter and disrupt the gut terrain at the microbial level. These imbalances can remain even after the medications have been discontinued.

It can be very difficult to resolve irritable bowel syndrome, food sensitivities, and microbial infections in the intestines and bowels due to a weakened or hypervigilant immune response, nervous system dysfunctions, slow or fast transit times, or a primary *Borreliosis* or *Bartonella* infection. All these factors must be considered in conjunction with emotional and psychological stress.

With persistent Lyme, advanced polymerase chain reaction (PCR) and culture testing is essential to rule out harmful overgrowth when experiencing ongoing gastric troubles despite dietary modifications. A food poisoning, non-acute overgrowth of harmful microbes, and translocation of different species of microbes from one part of the digestive tract to another can cause ongoing gastric troubles. Different microbes live in different parts of the gut in a healthy individual, where they maintain a unique and delicate homeostasis.

As Lyme and coinfection symptoms can activate suddenly, dietary choices and therapeutic modalities must be adjusted accordingly. Acute nutritional modifications can help calm down flare-ups and provide anti-inflammatory support. This requires careful dietary coaching on a weekly basis, especially during crisis mode. For some individuals with severe gastric distress, food choices initially can become extremely limited. It can be a challenge to ensure that the individual is not malnourished when multiple food eliminations, lack of absorption, and infections are in play.

Gut infections can trickle down into the urogenital tract, creating more uncomfortable and painful symptoms that mimic Lyme. Infections become embedded in the bladder, prostate, or urinary tract; thus, the multiple infections become a difficult puzzle to solve.

Major glands and organs involved in digestive challenges include the following:

- Hormones, mood chemicals, and immune cells in the gut are in constant communication with the hypothalamus, pituitary, and adrenals via the vagus nerve. Like a super highway, it connects to all organs and glands involved in the complex digestive process. This is the gut-brain axis.

- The thyroid gland plays an important role in peristalsis, a process by which involuntary muscle contractions move our ingested food onward through the digestive system. A hypothyroid condition must be considered with constipation.
- The kidneys are closely connected to the digestive system. With a lack of digestive power, kidney function is insufficient, which can result in water retention, toxic build up, increased uric acid levels, kidney stones, low electrolyte levels, or too frequent urination.
- The adrenal glands are our stress responders. With perceived stress there is decreased output of hydrochloric acid, increased blood sugar, and lowered immune protection in the gut.
- The spleen, according to Chinese medicine, is the seat of the immune system and rules the digestive system. The spleen and digestive system work together to increase digestive energy.
- The pancreas also shows signs of enzyme-secreting deficiency when the body is under tremendous stress. This contributes to blood sugar problems and indigestion, which can have far-reaching consequences in any part of the digestive tract.
- The liver stores glycogen, clears chemicals toxins and hormones, filters excess histamine, and cleans our blood.

Our digestive health is directly connected to our mood and sleep health. Neurotransmitters in the brain, including the feel-good and pain-killing chemicals, are made from amino acids in the foods we eat—if the gut is working well. The gut-brain connection is one of the reasons why selective serotonin reuptake inhibitor (SSRI) medications impact the digestive system.[1] (SSRIs are the most commonly prescribed antidepressants and include Lexapro, Prozac, Paxil, and Zoloft.)

Brain chemicals such as serotonin and melatonin are mostly made in the gut, not in the brain. An unhealthy gut will play a crucial role in all mood and sleep disorders, as will a toxic and inflamed brain.

This was already established over a hundred years ago by Nobel-recipient

Dr. Elie Metchnikoff, a pioneer in the field of intestinal microbes, probiotics in yogurt, and the relationship of toxins, including ammonia, phenols, and indols, in relationship to aging and mental health.[2] This whole health paradigm is continued by progressive psychiatrists, including Dr. Kelly Brogan in New York City, who are not afraid to challenge the long-term, commercial, hard-core (and business-driven) pharmaceutical treatment for mood and sleep disorders, which dismisses the scientific evidence regarding the impact of gut health, infections, and nutrition in mood disorders.

B12 deficiencies contribute to many symptoms that are similar to those of vector-borne infectious diseases, including anemia, dementia, depression, and cardiovascular, mental, and neurological challenges. A vitamin B12 deficiency is common in a vegetarian diet.[3] With compromised digestion and gut flora imbalances, it is difficult to produce sufficient levels of vitamin B12, which is separated from proteins in food in the body in the presence of hydrochloric acid. This is a complex process called the *intrinsic factor*. Stress, lack of rest, and infections suppress the parasympathetic nervous system that governs our digestion. This adversely affects the body's innate ability to produce a sufficient amount of stomach acid and thus vitamin B12. Consider how you can best optimize your digestion and have your doctor check your B12 and folic acid levels. But be aware that blood tests are not accurate because they measure the B12 levels in the bloodstream and not the active B12 availability inside the body's tissues.

Besides nutritional modifications and digestive aids, healing of the gut includes various herbal therapies, homeopathy, essential oils, acupuncture, glandulars, and chiropractic and craniosacral care. There are other healing arts that are supportive as well, including reflexology, energy medicine, massage, and BodyTalk. Meditation, deep-breathing exercises, and calming activities improve your digestion by targeting the vagus nerve, which activates the parasympathetic nervous system. These stress-reducing modalities support the individual from a whole-person perspective. It is about reconnecting the flow and communication between our cells, our heart, and our positive mind that supports our healing potential.

Our body wants us to be well.

Digestion—Or Is It Indigestion?

When we discuss the lengthy process of digestion, we must begin with mastication. From a mechanical perspective, we must chew our food well. This important but often neglected process induces the release of stomach acid, bile, and enzymes needed for digestion.

So, take your time and chew well. Feel how the tongue is involved in swirling motions and how your muscles work when you swallow. Chewing hard foods such as apples and carrots provide pumping action in the brain, which facilitates brain drainage. Allow meridians in your jaw and taste buds on your tongue to signal the brain, glands, vagus nerve, and organs that interconnect with digestive organs and glands. Chewing alerts them all of upcoming action. This is especially important if the vagus nerve is compromised by paralysis from the vector-borne infections.

Bitter foods and zinc are needed to stimulate the production of hydrochloric acid. It is protective and part of our immune system; the hydrochloric acid neutralizes harmful foodborne pathogens (such as parasites or salmonella) that enter our bodies through foods. This function is very important when dealing with persistent Lyme because the gut immune system is often already compromised.

Lack of stomach acid will slow the digestive process, creating a fertile feeding ground for opportunistic yeasts and bacteria along the tract. Stagnation of undigested food creates symptoms of indigestion, bloating, and acid reflux along the digestive tract. It has far-reaching effects that can include acne, hair loss, and weak fingernails.

Hydrochloric acid (with an optimal pH of one to three) is essential to facilitate the absorption of minerals and proteins from foods. Lack of stomach acid and digestive enzymes makes breaking down food difficult, especially proteins, and the food will rot and ferment in the stomach.

I recommend not drinking water or excessive liquids with meals. It dilutes hydrochloric acid into a more alkaline solution, which interferes with digestion.

Lack of stomach acid also adversely affects the trapdoor, the important esophageal sphincter that separates the stomach from the intestines. Dysfunction of the sphincter can result in backflow of undigested food and bile. That does not sound very good, and it certainly does not feel very good. If you think you might have a stomach ulcer, this must be ruled out by a physician. (This sphincter dys-regulation must also be considered with SIBO and an active *Helicobacter pylori* infection in the stomach that siphons away the stomach acid.)

Many people are not aware that putrefaction of foods, acid reflux, and gast-roparesis is often caused by a lack of stomach acid. Putrefaction of foods leads to too much acid production with burning discomfort. Commercial treatment includes acid-blocking medications such as proton pump inhibitors. Unfortu-nately, gastroenterologists usually prescribe long-term use of antacids that sup-press idiopathic gastrointestinal distress and reflux without investigating root causes.

Many respiratory and digestive troubles are interconnected because the esophagus and trachea are closely connected. If one is inflamed, so is the other. A persistent Lyme infection can make both worse. It is important to eliminate known food allergens, infectious agents, and environmental and chemical expo-sures that increase irritation and inflammation in the digestive and respiratory pathways.

Unfortunately, it can be difficult to connect digestive and respiratory symp-toms to ingested foods. Some adverse responses don't show until seventy-two hours after ingestion. And then, it might not be the food but the pesticides on the foods that are causing distress in the gut. In addition, different food combi-nations can have cross reactions, so you might not know which food gave you trouble. As an example, about fifty percent of individuals who are sensitive to gluten do not tolerate dairy. Other foods that cross-react with gluten include cof-fee, hemp, buckwheat, chocolate, yeast, sorghum, soy, teff, and whey. Antibody and cross-reaction testing by Cyrex labs is helpful for many, but it is expensive and not available in the state of New York.[4]

In an acute crisis of the gut, medications can absolutely help prevent serious consequences. However, in many cases, medications, such as for acid reflux, are prescribed for the long term without further investigation. That is a problem, a big problem. Acid-blocking medications adversely affect the absorption of proteins and minerals that are needed when dealing with chronic Lyme and mood disorders. It can result in low levels of zinc, magnesium, and calcium, cramping, muscle weak-ness, and bone and teeth problems. In certain cases, short-term pharmaceutical relief care can help prevent formation of ulcers and increased inflammation of the esophagus and stomach lining while root causes are investigated.

The use of any medications, especially over-the-counter pain medications, mood-altering medications, histamine blockers, opioids, and antibiotics, must also be considered when digestive stress is present. Short-or long-term use of medications irritate the stomach lining, especially pain medications, analgesics, and anti-inflammatories, which are often prescribed for Lyme-related joint pains. Antidepressant medications suppress an important enzyme that is needed to break down histamine. This matters for those with histamine-related symptoms, underlying anxiety, and most cell disorders. These have the potential to increase inflammation while also interfering with the diversity of the gut flora.

Digestive healing is a long-term process best done in conjunction with a knowledgeable nutrition specialist who sees the big picture and creates a simple-to-follow strategy for your needs. One must allow for flexibility as any additional stress input can create more disruption. Each individual has a unique history and microbiome blueprint with their own genetic factors and daily life challenges, so no two treatment protocols are the same. Persistent Lyme with digestive ailments is complex and advanced gut testing is recommended. The compromised body can be very reactive when it is pushed too far and too soon for what it can handle.

Digestive First-Aid: Enzymes

When it comes to digestive enzymes, there are plant-based enzymes and animal-sourced enzymes. Different digestive enzymes perform different functions. They are also sensitive to the varying pH levels in the different sections of the gut as well as your body temperature and your dietary choices. Enzymes are like construction workers; they break down proteins, carbohydrates, and fats in our foods into molecules that our body can absorb. These include pepsin, maltase, trypsin, chymotrypsin, and lipase. (Just to be very clear, I am discussing digestive enzymes, not the proteolytic enzymes that are used for biofilm disruption.)

Plant-based digestive enzymes are active within a broader range of pH levels in comparison to animal-sourced enzymes. They are primarily involved in breaking down vegetables and fruit fibers compared to animal-sourced enzymes that are more helpful with the breakdown of animal proteins. Check the sourcing of digestive enzymes; some can be sourced from soy, barley, pineapple, or papaya, which might not agree with you.

Animal-sourced digestive supplements come from pancreatic or stomach enzymes that are derived mostly from cows or pigs. These are strong metabolic enzymes; the pancreatin contains the enzymes proteases, amylases, and lipases that an optimally functioning pancreas would secrete. Choose brands such as Biotics Research, Thorne, Enzymedica, Designs for Health, MediHerb, and Standard Process that are mostly allergen-free. The addition of an unknown allergic burden in a supplement could make it even more difficult to isolate what is irritating your gut. Always discuss supplementation with a professional before adding them to your nutritional strategy.

To Juice or Not to Juice

Raw foods and juicing, while a great source of fiber and enzymes, can present challenges for many. Raw foods are cooling foods and are not going to be helpful for a weakened digestive system unless warming foods, such as ginger, are added. Instead, eat mostly cooked or prepared foods if you have gastric distress, which is prevalent with chronic illness, or if you are living in a cold climate. Juicing of lower-glycemic raw vegetables may be tolerated if you live in a hot climate, but it is certainly not recommended for all.

I recommend juicing selectively with blanched or steamed vegetables instead of raw vegetables. Keep in mind that juicing can be contraindicated for some individuals because the concentrated food form can bring on a severe detox.

To Ice or Not to Ice

It is best to avoid all iced and chilled drinks, smoothies, and ice cream. These will cause cramping and shut down food transit or gut motility, which in many cases is already compromised. Imagine what it feels like when you jump into an ice-cold pool. Your whole body contracts and shivers. This is what happens to your digestive tract when you drink iced water or drinks—it causes contraction, constriction, and constipation. Eating ice cream after a meal will also adversely affect the digestion of the just-eaten meal.

A much better option is to drink a warm liquid that increases circulation and prepares the digestive tract for incoming food. In a Chinese restaurant, you get warm tea before and after the meal that stimulates digestion. In most restaurants in the United States, you get iced water before your meal that shuts down digestion.

Whole Food Probiotics

With chronic Lyme infections, fermented vegetable juices and foods can help repopulate a healthy gut ecology. These traditionally prepared foods are nutrient-dense, high-fiber foods. The fermented vegetables are somewhat predigested, and thus more bioavailable, with a great source of vitamin C.

Unfortunately, fermented foods are no longer part of the standard diet, which is a loss for traditional gut healing. Cheeses, wines, sourdough bread, and yogurt left to sour all provide naturally fermented and enzyme-rich foods that has supported gut health for generations. Fermented or pickled foods were, and still are, part of many traditional diets. The bonus in fermented foods is not just in eating of the vegetable but also the consumption of the fermented liquid in the jar. Start with a small amount and see if you can tolerate it. It is best when enjoyed as part of a meal.

Many people with gut troubles and abdominal symptoms have difficulty with high-fiber vegetables, even though fermented foods provide a great source of gut-friendly bacteria and nutrients. Eating fermented vegetables at this time might not be an ideal food choice, yet ingesting the fermented juice from the vegetables might be tolerated. In some individuals, fermented foods can trigger bloating, headaches, and inflammation-related flare-ups. Histamine accumulation comes into play here, and various health, skin, respiratory, and psychotic problems are connected with elevated histamine levels in the blood. As the gut heals and flora is repopulated, traditionally fermented foods can hopefully be reintegrated. Genetic factors can also affect your ability to tolerate these foods. If you do not do well with fermented vegetables or juices at this time, eliminate them from your diet.

Leaky Gut Syndrome–A Gateway to Autoimmune Diseases

The gut lining is a big part of the inner defense system, just like a border patrol that keeps out the bad guys. The integrity and thickness of the mucosal lining is very important because it is the prime site for our immune response system to launch an assault against outside antigens. If the integrity of the intestinal lining is compromised, it opens the door for food-borne infections and toxins to gain access, which result in food sensitivities, malnutrition, skin problems, various inflammatory autoimmune conditions, and infections with systemic implications. We call this leaky gut syndrome; however, your physician will probably be more receptive to your concerns if you use the terminology *intestinal permeability*. Vitamin-rich foods, mucilaginous foods, spices, herbs, and gut-nourishing broth fortify this important fast-healing protective barrier.

Imagine the gut is like a bicycle tube that uses membranes to keep harmful agents and toxins out of our bodies. These membranes are an important part of our immune system. The moist membranes, which line our gut, nose, mouth, eyes, lungs, and urogenital tract, serve as barriers between the outside world and the inside of our body. Membranes in the gut play a large role in our ability to absorb essential nutrients from foods and to fight off harmful microbes that enter our bodies through food, such as parasites.

Now, imagine that the bicycle tube has small holes in it and the contents can spill into the bloodstream. This is what happens with a leaky gut when the gut membranes and finger-like villi structures open up, allowing entry for harmful pathogens and food molecules. Food molecules and toxins can now leak into the bloodstream, triggering an immune system response that is always coupled with inflammatory chemicals that harm our bodies. You can imagine how agitated and irritated the gut and the brain are when this takes place.

If you eat gluten-containing foods, the body will release a substance called *zonulin*. Zonulin, a naturally produced protein, regulates the permeability of the gut membranes; necessary substances can pass through the spaces, but harmful microbes are blocked when the integrity of membranes is not compromised. In the presence of gliadins, found in foods that contain gluten, and pesticides, especially glyphosate, the spaces open up wider—too wide. This allows larger molecules from foods, external infectious agents, and environmental toxins to get into our body. These are not supposed to pass through our protective membrane barrier. As a result, the immune system goes on high alert in an attempt to neutralize the foreign molecules in the blood stream or those that have settled on our joints or glands and mimic our own cells in a process called *molecular mimicry*. This immune and stress response is coupled with inflammation and will make all Lyme symptoms worse. Alcohol, emotional stress, medications, and concussions can induce a leaky gut, too, setting the scene for development of autoimmune diseases that can happen in any part of the body.

This can also occur in the blood-brain barrier, which is a protective screening barrier that separates the circulating blood from the brain, allowing nutrients into the brain and keeping toxins out. A leaky brain barrier results in an inflamed brain, which is implicated in autism spectrum disorders, sleep disorders, biotoxin illnesses, neurological diseases, concussions, and psychiatric symptoms.

Research shows that gluten-containing foods (and infections) can trigger neurological disorders that also mimic or worsen Lyme-related symptoms, even without the presence of a leaky gut. Gluten antibodies (and viruses) have been shown to increase cytokines. The release of these inflammatory chemicals is associated with immune activation. When the immune system detects the gluten antibodies (or Lyme spirochetes) in brain tissue or any other organ or gland, it perceives it as a threat and goes after it to destroy it. This causes tremendous inflammation in the brain, destruction of nerve tissue, and early degeneration of the brain.

In the United States, gluten sensitivity is rapidly on the increase; however, excessive processing of food, pesticide sprayings, exposure to poisonous glyphosate, and excessive consumption all must be considered. The question is this: Which component is driving an overactive immune response? Is it the stress that compromises the gut? Pesticides? Gluten? Infections? Or is it all of them together? Elimination of gluten is strongly recommended when living with vector-borne infections because of the multiple inflammatory factors previously mentioned.

With gut healing, key components include—

- Removal of offending foods, including gluten, refined sugars, yeast, and possibly dairy
- Digestive support, such as digestive enzymes, hydrochloric acid, or bitters
- Elimination of harmful microbes
- Repair of the gut lining
- Modulation of the immune system/consideration of histamine, oxalate and salicylate challenges
- Repopulation with diverse beneficial microbes (probiotics)
- Modulation of inflammation

The Lyme infection is not within your control, but if you can dial down the systemic inflammation and neurological damage associated with a leaky gut and gluten exposures, it can help alleviate your symptoms.

Antibodies in blood screenings are strong predictors of future autoimmune diseases. These appear far ahead of the development of symptoms and diagnosed pathology and thus can be considered an early warning sign. For example, thyroid antibodies can indicate future autoimmune challenges in the thyroid gland, or pancreatic antibodies can be future predictors of diabetes type 1. A leaky gut is a common denominator in all. More than eighty clinically distinct autoimmune diseases have been identified, and between five and eight percent of individuals are afflicted in the United States.[5]

Other causes of a leaky gut include—

- Stress
- Alcohol consumption
- Food poisoning
- Food intolerances
- GMOs
- Processed foods
- C-section birth
- Smoking
- Amalgam fillings

- Gastric infections
- Vaccinations
- Medications
- Gluten
- Surgery
- Antibiotics in foods
- Lifestyle choices
- Flu shots
- Emotional trauma
- Nervous system and brain support (including vagal nerve stimulation with slow transit difficulties)

Potential risk for autoimmune diseases cannot be based solely on genetic factors. Your genes are not your destiny. The impact of epigenetics (external factors that affect your genetic makeup) includes the interplay of diet, lifestyle, vaccinations, infections, heavy metal toxicity and atmospheric aluminum exposures, emotional stress, and multiple other toxic environmental influences in combination with existing genetic predispositions. All factors play an important role in our ability to become well again.[6] It is not only about Lyme disease. With a focus on individual gut health and digestive wellness, one can make targeted interventions to prevent continuation of the disease process while treating Lyme or other infections.

Lyme and Biofilm

Biofilm, a complex matrix of microorganisms in which cells stick to each other and often adhere to a surface, is a common occurrence in the human body and in nature. It can create a challenge for the immune system because harmful microbes can go undetected in biofilm or in cysts. In these protective structures, harmful pathogens evade antimicrobial treatment, including antibiotics. This contributes to persistent infections and relapses despite prior or current medical treatment. (Lyme spirochete and *Giardia* parasites favor cyst forms to ensure their survival in our body.) Biofilm in our body is mainly comprised of minerals from the foods we eat; thus, it can contribute to nutritional deficiencies of the host, including magnesium, calcium, and iron. In addition, carbs, fats, and proteins are taken directly from our bloodstream. Other components can include various metals we accumulate in our body. Biofilm and cysts enable the formation of persister cells that are a hallmark of ongoing infection and Lyme sickness.

The intricate matrix originates as part of a natural process when microbes attach to a living or nonliving surface. Biofilm includes health-supporting microbes in our mouth, nose, throat, and urogenital tract, even our appendix is a reservoir that is called upon with infections.[7] An immense array of microorganisms grow into self-contained microcolonies, forming a dynamic and protective matrix. Imagine this similar to a coral reef structure that forms a protective housing community or slime that is found on the surface of a pond and is filled with different types of algae. In contrast, biofilm with harmful microbes can include amyloid plaque in the brain associated with Alzheimer's, which encapsulates viral infections or plaque on the teeth. Biofilm also provides a home for infections that settle on titanium joint replacements or the pneumonia in cystic fibrosis or Candida infections in the urinary tract. It is also inside catheters, prosthetic heart valves, and tubes used in medical treatment, adding to medical complications.

Microbes are smart; they want to survive, communicate, and propagate. They are able to come and go as they please, and they hide in biofilm, cysts, or nerve and organ tissues when they sense that the environment is threatening their survival. They also hide in the lymphatic system, where antibiotic treatment and herbal therapies cannot get to them.

As part of their natural life cycle, harm-inducing microbes excrete poisonous waste within channels of the biofilm, and these endotoxins contribute to many symptoms of sickness. They also become more aggressive when they feel threatened, releasing more toxins as self-defense.

In addition, lipopolysaccharides (LPS) are also present. These are released from the membranes of gram negative bacteria that can cause a lot of trouble if not kept in check. LPS triggers a localized immune and inflammatory response, which can result in a systemic infection causing sepsis and septic shock. Manifestations of localized involvement can be bronchitis, cystitis, or inflammatory diarrhea. This occurs when the immune system recognizes LPS in the mucosa of the gastrointestinal, urinary, and respiratory tract. The presence of LPS is another factor to consider with vector-borne infections.

Microbes exchange DNA, recruit other microbes, and communicate with each other in a self-organizing process called *quorum sensing*, which is similar to the way bees and ants communicate with each other in nature. In order to get rid of harmful microbes and Lyme spirochetes or round forms (a shape spirochetes use to evade the immune system) in the body, biofilm and cysts must be broken down with specific protein-based enzymes, stevia, or herbal or homeopathic formulas such as guggul.

Protein enzymes include nattokinase, lumbrokinase, Boluoke, Interfase Plus, or serrapeptase. But, it is essential to initiate lymphatic drainage before treating biofilm and infections. There is no point in attacking microbes when the body cannot get rid of the debris and the channels of elimination and detoxification are blocked. This will result in a herx once treatment is started and can make you feel and think that you are getting worse.

The body must be able to clean the fluid between the cells where toxins and infections reside. Internal house cleaning must occur on a regular basis and it mostly happens at night when we are asleep. During sleep, the body has time to pay attention to clearing toxins, especially the dumping of toxic waste from the brain. If one cannot sleep, this detox and lymphatic drainage do not occur. Toxins accumulate and increase inflammation. All psychiatric, behavioral, cognitive, and other Lyme symptoms will become worse, including excessive fatigue that prevents you from getting out of bed.

Plus, any integrated biofilm-breaking approach must include the addition of bile salts, anti-inflammatory herbs, binding agents (e.g., chlorella, charcoal, or bentonite), immune-modulating herbals or homeopathics, and adrenal stress support. Epsom salt baths, acupuncture, and ionized foot baths are also very helpful in minimizing die-off reactions that can occur.

A special note: If biofilm-breaking agents and antimicrobials are used to combat biofilm in gastro-intestinal infections, it will affect Lyme-related biofilm and cyst infections. Caution is advised. Proteolytic (protein-based) enzymes and antimicrobials can interfere with Lyme treatment, increasing herx reactions, pain, and systemic inflammation. If you are in treatment, you do not want to do anything that interferes with your Lyme or coinfection treatment. Discuss this with your doctor. If you are not in active treatment but have Lyme-related symptoms, do not start any supplementation without appropriate professional guidance.

THE SIBO AND LYME DILEMMA

Root causes of small intestinal bacterial overgrowth (SIBO) can be associated with Lyme-associated infections, antibiotics, hypothyroidism, accidental food poisoning, brain injuries, physical abnormalities, a diet high in carbohydrates with refined sugars, psycho-emotional stress, lack of stomach acid, and surgeries. These factors can cause or contribute to an impaired digestive system, allowing for translocation of microbes through various parts of the digestive tract and altered nerve function in the bowels. Common symptoms associated with SIBO include post-meal bloating, indigestion, abdominal pain around the navel, hemorrhoids, bad breath, acid reflux, constipation or diarrhea (or both), and foul-smelling gas. It is not just about Lyme disease.

Bacteria from the colon do not belong in the small intestine. When the natural sweeping action in the bowels is compromised, it allows certain bacteria (even health-supporting ones) from the colon to migrate upward to the small intestine. Use of certain probiotics and prebiotics can make these symptoms worse. Fermentation of high-fiber foods in the bowels then occurs with the release of toxic gases, including methane and hydrogen.

High-fiber foods include legumes, alliums, cruciferous vegetables, grains, and fruits. SIBO recipe websites as a resource might be helpful, and remember to customize your food choices according to what you can tolerate and digest.

Lyme infections that target and paralyze nerves in the digestive tract and ongoing oral antibiotic treatment for Lyme are a challenge with SIBO. How severely symptoms manifest is unique to each individual. Multiple strategies must be implemented at the same time to optimize the pH and encourage functions of various organs and glands in the digestive tract, while shifting the ecology in the gut towards wellness. With SIBO and Lyme, difficulties with gastric emptying can also occur, including a challenging condition called *gastroparesis* that requires nutritional modifications. At all times, the resilience and strength of the host must be fortified to withstand an attack from opportunistic yeasts. This requires a customized nutritional approach with appropriate food preparations and additional digestive support.

It is important to consider the terrain in which the SIBO/SIFO infection was allowed to flourish. Any food poisoning, abdominal surgery, excessive inflammation, psychological or emotional trauma, or Lyme-related infections can impair the nerves that are in charge of sweeping waste materials through the intestines. This neurologically driven mechanism is known as *intestinal motility* or the *migrating motor complex*, and it is closely connected to the brain. Dietary modifications are only successful if the brain and the nervous system are included in treatment of SIBO.

If the brain is on fire with vector-borne infections and toxins, the connection between the brain and the gut will be compromised. Infections and their toxins present difficult challenges because they paralyze the enteric nervous system (the system that governs the function of the gastrointestinal system), including the vagus nerve. It is very perceptive and can sense when, for instance, the brain is inflamed or a Lyme infection or a herpes virus is in play.

The vagus nerve is the longest nerve in the body; it runs down most of our torso. It is closely connected to the esophagus, stomach, spleen, lungs, and brain, and, simply put, it affects various organs and glands that are consequential to our wellness. The vagus nerve is involved in the release of enzymes, blood flow to the intestines, and intestinal motility (migrating motor complex). Stress, inflammation, and infections directly impact this nerve and, thus, affect the function of all the organs and glands. With Lyme-induced paralysis, vagal nerve dysfunction presents a very difficult situation as it is also closely related with blood pressure swings, such as in POTS. The vagus nerve must be retrained in its activation to allow for improved transit in the digestive tract.

According to Lyme expert, Dr. Dietrich Klinghardt, it is important to initially offload the function of the vagus nerve so that it can heal while underlying vector-borne and gastric infections are being treated. Off-loading the nerve includes modifying nutrition and adding digestive aids including hydrochloric acid before each meal.

If your mind is stressed, the gut is stressed. Consider that the gut is actually like a second brain with its own nervous system, the enteric nervous system. But the nervous system in the brain and the enteric nervous system are in constant communication. Of the roughly one hundred million nerves in your gut, between one thousand and two thousand nerves are communicating with the brain. Any thought, mental stress, or internal or external challenges will affect our digestive loop, which begins in the mouth and ends with the anus.

Picture the nerve pathways as being like a superhighway between the brain and bowels, with traffic flowing in both directions all day every day. You can imagine how an accident on a Los Angeles highway creates traffic problems, backing up traffic for miles and creating chaos. Imagine this dysfunctional scenario in the human body when the gut-brain connection is not working well or there is nerve damage in the intestines. We must reestablish communication.

If you have certain microbial overgrowth in the small intestine, initially avoid probiotics that contain prebiotic fiber, including insulin, chicory root, or fructooligosaccharides (FOS). They can cause bloating and gas if there is unwelcome microbial overgrowth in the intestines. It is concerning to eliminate prebiotic fiber from the diet for too long because it will affect the microflora and the production of butyrate, which are important when living with Lyme.

Gastrointestinal motility can be encouraged with the herbal formulas Iberogast or MotilPro. There is more information regarding the gut-brain connection and motility in chapter nine. Overall stress, including emotional and psychological stress, and hormonal imbalances, including adrenal insufficiency, must be considered too; treatment must be addressed from all angles, from a whole-person perspective. Going on a bug-killing spree with rifaximin for diarrhea and hydrogen dominant IBS or SIBO will not prevent a relapse of SIBO if underlying imbalances are not resolved. Antratil is gathering great interest for constipation—methane dominant SIBO or IBS.

Methane and hydrogen are the main players in SIBO, yet a breath test can be negative, even though a SIBO condition is present with clinical findings. Biofilm structures and yeast overgrowth are part of this complex scenario. Small intestinal fungal overgrowth (SIFO) is the latest addition. This has been known as *dysbiosis* in the past; however, the incidences and diagnosis of SIBO is greatly increasing. SIBO or dysbiosis can be considered with—

- Abdominal pain, nausea, heartburn, acid reflux, bloating, belching, and severe gas
- Constipation (especially with methane gas), diarrhea, or a combination of both
- Malabsorption of nutrients, including iron, vitamin K, and vitamin B12 (with or without anemia)
- Impaired detoxification in the liver
- Lactose intolerance
- Increased fatigue
- Bad breath
- Skin problems, such as rosacea or idiopathic skin eruptions
- Increased pain with increased inflammation
- Mood disorders—depressed moods and anxiety
- Sleep disturbances caused by decreased melatonin production
- Thyroid, adrenal, and sex hormone imbalances including PMS, cysts, and low testosterone
- Autoimmune diseases such as Crohn's and interstitial cystitis

It is interesting to note that vector-borne infections also cause all of these symptoms. Lyme is, after all, called the great imitator.

With active Lyme-related symptoms or use of antibiotics and other medications, it can be difficult to make desired progress—but it is possible if a modified diet is adhered to. It is a long-term process that is different for each individual, and I will be frank: It is not easy. Elimination of SIBO (and SIFO) takes an integrated approach with strict dietary measures. Dietary approaches include a variation of the low FODMAP foods, the Specific Carbohydrate Diet, Auto-Immune Diet, and the Gut And Psychology Syndrome diet (GAPS). In severe cases, there is a three-week elemental diet that must be done with professional supervision.

SIBO is often treated with pharmaceutical agents, including antibiotics, low-dose naltrexone (LDN), and bowel motility–supporting medications called *prokinetics.* In many cases, the infection returns or the drug therapy is not effective, especially if dietary modifications are not implemented, and the overall immune system remains challenged by other underlying infections. Treating SIBO, and preventing relapses, requires treating the person as a whole.

Tests are available for SIBO that can be done at a physician's office (involving a lactulose breath test to discern hydrogen and methane gas after ingesting a specific solution). There are also tests available that you can do at home. However, some individuals cannot tolerate or afford these tests, and some give false-negative results despite fungal or SIBO-like symptoms. An easy and inexpensive self-test is to make a soup from vegetables on the high FODMAP food list and see how your body responds. If your symptoms worsen and you experience severe gassiness, bloating, or bowel activity changes, you will know that there is an underlying bacterial overgrowth concern.

Eradication of harmful bacteria in the small intestine has been found to alleviate symptoms associated with fibromyalgia, psychiatric illness, and Lyme infections, yet this is not considered in commercial medicine.

There is never just one infection; we must think broader. When there is trouble in one part of the digestive system, there are also challenges in other parts of the digestive tract. All are concomitant with a leaky gut and with Lyme (and prolonged antibiotic use), and that is an ongoing concern. Symptoms can also occur in other parts of the body. Thus, if there is an idiopathic skin problem, such as atopic dermatitis, it is very unlikely that the commercially trained dermatologist will consider the leaky gut or a possible fungal or SIBO infection. They will likely give you a steroid cream or some other pharmaceutical as treatment.

If there are no satisfactory improvements despite food eliminations and antimicrobial treatment for intestinal bacterial overgrowth, think big picture. A comprehensive digestive stool analysis from a specialized lab that tests specimens at a genetic level can be helpful in identifying additional infections in the lower bowels. Other pathogens such as parasites, worms, and fungi can add a burden on the immune system. These can be hidden infection such as tapeworms or hookworms and can prevent a SIBO infection, and Lyme, from clearing.

Keep in mind that no test is a hundred percent foolproof. Stool tests can give insight into twenty-four commensal bacteria and identify various pathogens using a highly specialized technology that amplifies trace amounts of DNA. This testing is also used for Lyme and coinfection diagnosis. It is called *polymerase chain reaction testing* (PCR). However, some harmful microbes are hiding higher up in the intestines or inside organs. Some parasites might be in cyst form, or they may avoid detection in biofilm. (This also happens with chronic Lyme and coinfections.)

There are many treatment options for SIBO. If you have it, you must decide what is best for you. Often, a cocktail of herbs and biofilm busters work well; however, it is also important to rotate herbals to avoid resistance (just like antibiotics—after all, herbs are antibiotic). Please note that if you have low blood sugar and low cholesterol, berberine might not be an optimal choice because it lowers blood sugar and cholesterol levels. Herbal applications are highly effective because they have a broad-spectrum influence on the immune, neurological, and hormonal level, and they support the body in many ways that we do not yet understand. Examples include St. John's wort, one of my favorites, which is an antiviral and an antidepressant; it also helps with sleep.

Nonpharmaceutical antimicrobial interventions can include neem, berberine, ginger, oregano oil, red thyme oil, garlic, Japanese knotweed, cat's claw (not the whole food form), artemesia, and professional products including Lauricin, Bacteria-Chord, Wormwood Complex, Gut Flora Complex, FC-Cidal, Dysbiocide, Cat's Claw Complex, goldenseal, and colostrum. Be sure to consult a health-care professional before taking any of these.

Herbals, just like antibiotics, also kill the health-supporting microbes in the gut. Use of certain probiotics is helpful in supporting the defense system in the gut. Probiotics that can be helpful include the spores in MegaSporeBiotic, or VSL-3, or *Lactobacillus plantarum*. *S. boulardii* is also helpful in many cases because it crowds out harmful yeasts that are commonly in play with SIBO. Others respond well to soil-based probiotics. Most importantly, probiotics can aid you in your current struggles with chronic Lyme. That is what really matters.

During antimicrobial treatment, eat moderate to high FODMAPS foods that call harmful microbes out of their hiding places. They get excited with high FODMAP foods and come out of hiding places to feed. That is when antimicrobial treatment is applied. Just like harm-inducing parasites or *H. pylori* in the digestive tract, you have to trick them to eradicate them.

We must also thin the bile, which is an important channel of our detoxification pathway. Thick, sludgy bile can result in gallstones, bloating, reflux, back pain, and inflammation. Radishes, beets, and beet tops are foods that thin the bile. Lyme infections, the accumulation of environmental toxins and chemical estrogens, medications, and sticky commercial fats create sludgy bile and increase the risk of gallstone formation. Using birth control pills is an additional challenge to the gallbladder.

Pharmaceutical treatment of SIBO involves antibiotic treatment, such as rifaxamin, or triple antibiotic treatment. Low-dose naltrexone and low-dose erythromycin are also often prescribed, yet not tolerated by all.

I am very concerned about the impact of antibiotics on the microbiome, cell membranes, and mitochondria in our cells. Antibiotics are overprescribed, but I know that certain physicians are judicious in their use. I will admit that some cases are very challenging and might respond better to an integrative approach. (Colonics and enemas must be part of the treatment program to prevent autointoxication.) Choose what is best for you.

How long it takes to get rid of SIBO and how symptomatic one is depends entirely on the individual. I have found dietary modifications with protein enzymes, hydrochloric acid, probiotics, and multiple rotations of herbal therapies effective. It takes time and patience, especially if the nervous system in the gut is disabled. You must continue to support the immune system, hormones, and gut flora to prevent a relapse.

The Fungal Dilemma

In nature, fungi and yeasts provide immune protection and decompose matter into nutrients for plants to absorb, or they create mushrooms for animals to eat. In the soil, their toxins are used by growing plants as antibiotics against other harmful pathogens. Yet if a plant is weakened by nutrient-deficient soil or a lack of water or sun, then harmful fungal overgrowth can occur; the fungus ends up eating the plant. It is the same in our gut. Yeasts and fungi are part of the healthy soil in our gut ecology. If the gut flora is diverse, the immune system is vigilant and modulated well, stress is reduced, and the host is well nourished, it creates a difficult environment for fungal infections to proliferate.

However, with persistent Lyme the host's immune function is weakened and digestion and hormones are challenged. Innate microbial checks and balances are off-kilter, especially with prolonged antibiotic and medication use. Herpes and stealth retroviruses suppress the immune system. With a weakened immune system, the individual is more vulnerable to pathogenic yeast, fungal overgrowth, and toxic mold exposures.

The toxins released from fungal infections such as gliotoxins from Candida or Aspergillus fumigates are powerful, and they contribute to many symptoms that mimic Lyme, including brain fog, neurological problems, insomnia, and systemic inflammation. In addition, Lyme expresses itself differently in various stages of the disease progression.

Addressing fungal infections is a double-edged sword. The fungal infection is opportunistic, but it can also have a deeper protective function. This can be viewed as a controversial perspective. Fungi and yeasts encapsulate toxic substances, heavy metals, and harmful microbes in the biofilm to protect us—yet the toxins released by the yeast and fungi infections, especially with threadlike growth in the body, harm us. They are very sensitive to their environment, including stress. When we get stressed, pathogens get stressed too. They become more active or release more toxins.

When working toward the eradication of fungal, Lyme-related, and other kinds of stealth infections, the additional toxic fallout must be considered. Fungal infections propagate in biofilm. When that is disrupted with chelating agents such as ethylenediaminetetraacetic acid (EDTA), proteolytic enzymes, or herbal formulations, the entrapped toxins, heavy metals, and microbes are released. This creates health problems for the host, especially if there are low levels of glutathione, sluggish bile, and constipation. The body cannot metabolize and eliminate the newly released toxins, and a herx reaction occurs that is not caused by the Lyme.

The adrenal glands, kidneys, gallbladder, and mitochondria must also be supported because they play a very important role in this process. Nutrients must be increased for energy at a cellular level. Glutathione supplementation must be part of the protocol when heavy metals are mobilized by killing yeasts, mold, and fungal infections in the body. It is essential to add binders that hold on to released metals and toxic waste so they do not get reabsorbed. If constipation is a symptom, it must be remedied to prevent auto-intoxication.

As you can see, multiple channels of elimination must be optimized to prevent extreme herx reactions that can, in severe cases, result in an emergency visit to the hospital. The above must be done with professional guidance or a Lyme-literate doctor.

Powerful Probiotics

I strongly recommend gut flora supplementation at any age to provide additional support for the gut flora. Customized therapeutic support has been helpful in alleviating various symptoms, including easing bloating and diarrhea and resolving constipation. There is great controversy regarding the use and effectiveness of probiotics. In my clinical experience, the introduction of soil-based probiotics and therapeutic high dosages of various probiotic strains and spores have been effective in easing various symptoms and increasing food tolerance. How probiotics affect the gut flora is different for each one of us because we each have a different gut microbe blueprint. My clients with infants have also experienced favorable results, especially with digestive ailments and regurgitation of food. Probiotics are imperative if a C-section birth and formula-feeding occurred.

Spores that survive the harsh gastric tract and support immune modulation are found in MegaSporeBiotic. This product has been very helpful in increasing tolerance of foods and decreasing allergies. Support with a healthy yeast species such as *S. boulardii* is beneficial in many cases, especially with bacterial overgrowth and fungal infections in the bowels—or thrush in the mouth, with localized application. Be aware that die-off reactions may occur with the introduction of probiotics and that it can make you feel worse, especially if constipation is a symptom. Yet probiotics can ease constipation for some. Everyone is different.

At present, there are multitudes of probiotics on the market, all claiming various benefits. I would consult with a health-care practitioner because the various strains, amounts, and bioavailability are important, especially if you are already experiencing severe abdominal symptoms. Intolerance to probiotics can occur;

this can be indicative of an inflammatory gut issue, which must be investigated, or a histamine-related reaction.

When it comes to probiotics, several questions must be considered:

- There are so many combinations possible; how do we know which probiotics are best for each individual's unique blueprint? There is no one right answer to that question because we do not know the many strains that make up our gut microbiome. However, a lack of bifidia strains can be implicated with lowered immune function.

- Probiotics are often stored in a fridge or freezer packed to protect them against warmer temperatures, yet the ideal body temperature is 98.6 degrees; does that not destroy the probiotics as they enter the body? Other probiotics and spores are not stored in a fridge. The discussions and research are ongoing.

- Where in nature does super dosing occur? Nowhere, and no study to date has shown the effectiveness of super dosing, yet clinical and anecdotal findings show lessening of symptoms for many.

- Do probiotics survive the journey through the upper gastrointestinal system with a strongly acidic pH? Probiotics stored in a cold environment are alive in the bottle, but they die when passing through the harsh pH digestive tract. This is controversial because some companies indicate that their product survives the harsh gastric transit. The debate continues.

- Only in childbirth and breastfeeding does a natural microbial inoculation and immune support in breast milk occur for the baby, just as nature intended. Are probiotics effective or a waste of money? Traditionally, fermented foods provided gut flora support, and exposures to dirt in nature have provided childhood and adult inoculations of soil-based bacteria. Our urban and sterilized lifestyles have altered our gut flora, and probiotics are one option to compensate for the natural inoculation. It is best to rotate multiple strains to increase diversity. Probiotics can help buffer the pH in the gut and ease digestive ailments and yeast-related symptoms.

These questions are certainly food for thought and, frankly, a rationale can be made for any argument. Though we will have to wait for more science on probiotics, current clinical and anecdotal findings do support probiotic applications in most cases. If you have children, let them play and eat dirt. If you have a garden, go and play with the dirt. That is a natural inoculation.

Probiotic vaginal, nasal washes, and rectal suppositories may be a more direct line into localized infections because they do not have to travel through the digestive tract. Tissues in these areas are highly sensitive and have a high absorption rate. This can be helpful with heavy metal chelation and antimicrobial treatment.

Fecal transplantations in clostridium difficile infections, have been effective. Think of it as a soil transplant—in effect, a microbiome transplant. However, there is an increased occurrence of autoimmune conditions after the transplant. Could this be connected with a leaky gut, or is it an immunological resistance to the introduction of foreign DNA? We will have to wait for more scientific findings on that matter.

With chronic Lyme, consideration of your gut flora diversity is helpful, and I firmly believe in supplementation. If it works for you that is great—that's all that matters.

. . . .

Wrapping Up

It is in the gut that we return to an innate source of mind-body nourishment. When living with Lyme infections, there are so many challenges that you deal with every day. With additional troubles in the digestive tract during active Lyme treatment or post-treatment, it is difficult to tend to daily tasks because of lack of energy and comfort.

My goal in this chapter is to provide you with insight into the various challenges that might be affecting you right now and why it is so important to tend to your gut health and digestive wellness. Lyme and other infections disturb the terrain, they can switch on dormant disease processes in the body, and they increase inflammation; this has a far-reaching effect. Whether you are on antibiotic treatment or not, your gut will be affected adversely at some point, if you are not already having digestive troubles. It is important to remember that our gut is our center. It affects our brain, immune system, energy, sex hormones, blood sugar balance, and mental outlook. If our gut is not well, no part in our body is well. If you are sick and do not know where to begin, start by taking care of your digestion, gut lining, and gut ecology, as outlined in the next chapter.

Yes, we are what we eat.

But it is also true that "we are what we, and our hundred trillion microbes, assimilate."

> "The doctor of the future will give no medication, but will interest
> his patients in the care of the human frame, diet, and in the cause
> and prevention of disease."
>
> —THOMAS EDISON

Chapter Eight

Action Steps to Optimize Digestion and Absorption

Pick one of the action steps below and start working on it today. It takes practice, but you will get better, and it will become part of your lifestyle.

1. It All Begins with a Shopping List

Plan ahead for shopping trips; make a list, and purchase foods that you can store in your cabinet and freezer. If you live in the city, there are grocery delivery options available that might be helpful and save you time and energy.

Start reading the labels of foods you enjoy. As you read the ingredients, see if you know what all the ingredients mentioned on the food label are. It might take more time to shop, but you will come out ahead by paying attention to what is in the food you are purchasing. The fewer ingredients listed on a food label, the better. Sometimes the first three ingredients are sugars, but they are listed with different names to disguise what they really are. Real foods with lots of energy and vitality have the least amount of ingredients. If you do not know an ingredient or cannot pronounce it, consider it a nonfood.

Even when buying in the organic section, look at the food labels. Ingredients are billed from the highest amount to the lowest. If the first ingredient is sugar, even if it is organic, cane, or coconut sugar, you might want to rethink your choice.

Foods with colors or additives are no-nos. All of these irritate and inflame the gut and brain. They also increase susceptibility to a leaky gut and food sensitivities. Here's a tip: Organic produce always has a nine in front of the other numbers on the sticker.

Become aware of how monosodium glutamate (MSG) can be hidden in food labels. There are over forty ingredients in processed foods that contain MSG, under the names hydrolyzed vegetable protein, soy protein isolate, and yeast extract, to name a few. It must only be labeled as MSG on the container if it contains ninety-nine percent pure MSG.

I also urge caution with organic flavored foods that contain added natural flavors such as vanilla, orange, or caramel. The sourcing of these flavors is often questionable, and they can irritate the body and brain. Cinnamon can also be an irritant for some individuals. Keep in mind that various added flavors are abundant in the food supply today, even in herbal teas. The following are some tips to remember when shopping:

- Avoid foods that just claim to be *natural* because the FDA has no guidelines for this term. Stay away from these foods.
- Refrain from synthetic flavors, such as vanilla, hazelnut, or pumpkin flavors used in drinks or yogurt.
- Steer clear of chemical colorants in foods and drinks.
- Educate yourself about various MSG names (look online) and avoid them as best you can.
- Preservatives in foods, including citric acid, can trigger an immune response. Stay with freshly prepared foods.
- Watch out for spices, especially spice packets in boxed rice and spices added to canned foods or soups. These spices will not be organic and will most likely contain large amounts of processed salt or MSG.

If possible, connect with farmers at markets and eat produce and fruits that are in season, unless you have the option to grow vegetables in your own garden. Foods that have no food label or expiration date on them are the best option (e.g., a bunch of radishes, yams, or marrow bones from the farmers' market). Seasonal produce and fruit that has been picked for the market will have the highest nutrient value. Many commercial foods are picked before they are ripe, and they ripen (or rot) during transportation. By the time they end up on our plate, the nutrient value is highly diminished.

2. Optimize Food Preparation

How you prepare your food matters greatly, especially when you and your body are very tired. Food preparation will make it easier for your body to take in the nutrients that it needs.

For basic food prep, you need a sieve, a steaming device (get a few different sizes, depending on which veggies you are steaming), a strainer, and a good blender. A crockpot or slow cooker is very economical and easy to use.

An important side note for toxin-free food prep is to avoid all nonstick cookware (and sprays) and invest in green cooking utensils. It is best to store foods in glass containers because plastic containers can leach chemical estrogens into the food, especially when heated.

Food preparation can be time-consuming if you have stomach troubles, but by putting forth the effort you can take steps toward changing ailments.

I recommend "pre-digesting" foods by steaming, stewing, blanching, baking, poaching, roasting, sautéing, slow cooking or slow grilling. Food can then be placed into a blender for further breakdown before it ends up on your plate (or in your bowl, if puréed). If your symptoms are severe, I recommend straining the puréed foods through a sieve for a low-fiber, baby food texture. Broth is a key dietary component in these cases because it is well tolerated and easy to digest. Steamed vegetables can be puréed and strained into a delicious broth. It is time-consuming, but with certain digestive concerns (e.g., SIBO or gastroparesis), this therapeutic approach is essential to improve tolerance for foods and absorption of nutrients.

With digestive challenges, high-protein animal food sources are easier to digest if you grind them up. If you do not have a grinder at home, ask the butcher to do it for you when you make your purchase at the store. Farmers' markets often have prepacked ground beef, lamb, turkey, or bison. Another option is ground chicken. You can create small patties of the protein of your choice, bound with cooked quinoa (instead of breadcrumbs). It is best to cook meats longer using lower temperatures to prevent destruction of nutrients, especially the B vitamins and heat-sensitive fats. A slow cooker or crockpot that requires minimum effort will provide you with many options.

After an initial period, when digestive troubles are resolved, you can hopefully return to consuming whole foods without excessive food preparation. From my experience, digestive enzymes, hydrochloric acid, and oxbile are very helpful when implementing a transition strategy.

Use of the microwave is best avoided because it alters the protein structure and cell wall structure of foods and liquids. (However, you can put your kitchen sponge in the microwave to get rid of the nasty bugs in the sponge!) The stovetop is your best friend.

3. Use Whole Foods to Heal Your Gut and Gut Lining

In my holistic practice, I use foods that support a leaky gut while also considering hidden food triggers. Mucilaginous plants, such as okra and aloe vera, and slimy foods, such as oatmeal or creamed buckwheat, support the gut lining. Learning which foods can help heal is always a better option than relying on lifelong supplementation. Let's focus on other foods that contain important nutrients for healing of the mucosal barrier.

Animal foods and shellfish contain the bioavailable form of vitamin A (and vitamin D). Cod liver oil is another great source of vitamin A. The mucosal linings, which line your lungs as well as your intestines, require vitamin A and vitamin C complex. Our eyes also need a great amount of vitamin A.

Beta-carotene is one of the carotenoid pigments in yellow, orange, and red vegetables and fruits. Some good sources are sweet potatoes, carrots, butternut squash, dark leafy vegetables, dried apricots, and papaya. They provide an array of phytonutrients and antioxidants that support the gut and overall health. However, beta-carotene must be converted in the body into vitamin A, and that conversion is a challenge for many individuals, who would do better ingesting the formed vitamin A found in animal foods, including eggs and butter (if tolerated).

Zinc is a key component for the immune system and connective tissues, including our skin, thyroid, bones, retinas, and gut membranes. It is also a key mineral that supports the gut lining, and we need it to produce stomach acid. Zinc is in a bioavailable form in animal, poultry, shellfish, and wild fish sources; yet with poor digestion, infections, and chronic stress, we deplete our zinc stores rapidly, causing a deficiency. White spots on your fingernails can indicate a zinc deficiency.

In legumes and dark leafy greens, phylates and oxalates can bind zinc, and the body is not able to unlock the bound form. This is why food preparation and cooking these particular vegetables is so important. Ideally, you should soak legumes in a bowl of water with a tablespoon of raw apple cider vinegar for at least twenty-four hours before cooking.

A pyrrole disorder might be in play with many individuals, and this can affect the ability to maintain optimal zinc levels. This underlying issue can hamper gut healing (and Lyme treatment), and in these cases, higher therapeutic dosages of zinc, vitamin B6, and other nutrients are needed *initially*.

Beware: Too much zinc is toxic, harms the immune system, and creates a disproportionate ratio with copper that creates other immune, hormonal, and neurological problems. The body has its own checks and balances: Every mineral, just like hormones and vitamins, works in conjunction with others. Yet sometimes there is need for a short-term therapeutic higher dose to overcome severe deficiencies.

Vitamin C is a water-soluble nutrient that is not stored in the body, so we regularly have to eat colorful foods rich in vitamin C daily to replenish our stores. Any chronic illness increases our need for vitamin C because the immune system, adrenal glands, and recycling of glutathione, our major antioxidant, depend on it. Foods rich in the whole vitamin C complex, not just the ascorbic acid, with its various cofactors and phystonutrients (as Mother Nature intended) include oranges, papaya, rosehips, kale, cauliflower, peppers, pineapple, kiwi, brussels sprouts, dark leafy greens, and parsley.

When cooking, it is best not to use a large amount of water because the water-soluble nutrients in foods, including vitamin C, leach into the water. Also, reduce cooking time to preserve more nutrients. Steaming is a better option, because more nutrients will be retained in the foods.

4. Support Healthy Gut Flora with Whole Foods and Fiber

Eating a variety of whole foods from organic, wild, and free-range sources and avoiding processed foods is the first line of defense. Rotating foods that support the diversity of the gut flora is the second line of defense. Maintaining a healthy flora in the bowels is crucial to facilitate competitive exclusion of harmful overgrowth and to protect against translocation of microbes that travel from the colon into the small intestine. Our gut flora is an integral part of the microbiome and is also called a *dynamic organ* and an *invisible organ*.[1] With fungal infections, elimination of dairy, grains, and high-glycemic foods is best.

Certain whole foods such as cultured milk and fermented foods such as Japanese natto and miso contain natural probiotics that support our inner gut ecology and women's vaginal ecology. Modern baking and processing practices, like adding yeasts, sugars, and other ingredients that are difficult to digest to foods, is very different from the way foods were fermented in traditional cultures.

Fermented foods, if they are fermented in the traditional way and do not contain alcohol, can also be considered predigested foods that are rich in vitamins and enzymes and support the gut flora. Foods such as sauerkraut, Kimchi, organic stoneground grains, and sourdough bread can be health supporting. These foods do not contain yeast or sugars if they are prepared in the traditional manner. The lactic acid process, which is naturally occurring, will break down grains and foods into bioavailable and nutrient dense foods. The culturing process with dairy products produces lactic acid that lowers the pH in the colon and urinary tract. A low pH in the stomach, colon, and vaginal tract is essential to ward off proliferation of harmful species, including *C. difficile* infections and yeast infections that are a concern common with prolonged antibiotic use.

It is important to remember that we are all different and that with Lyme-associated infections and treatments, the gut flora is often compromised and the immune system is less tolerant of various foods, especially high-histamine foods. Fermented foods can cause histamine or aldehyde-related symptoms, including headaches, itchy skin, and fatigue. I recommend starting with very small amounts and increasing by tiny increments to see if you can tolerate them.

Eating fiber-rich foods (soluble and insoluble) is the foundation for supporting your gut health, blood sugar, stool formation, and detoxification. The digestible fiber we eat in vegetables and fruits is a broad-spectrum prebiotic—probiotics ferment the fiber and produce short-chain fatty acids, or butyrate. Butyrate is very important when you are living with any persistent Lyme or mold infection. Cooked and cooled potatoes, a wide variety of fruits and vegetables, cooked and cooled rice and legumes, and dehydrated plantain chips all provide prebiotic value. (The cooking temperature of the food must be below 130 degrees to be beneficial.)

Polyphenols, as found in fruits, vegetables, red wine, olives, and tea leaves, also impact health-supporting microbes. This might be a carry over from our hunter-gatherer days with an adaption in our microbiome. They also encourage the health of the intestinal and urinary tract.

5. Let Us Not Forget about the Gallbladder and Liver

Healthy fats are essential for good health. But can you digest and absorb the fats you eat? Sometimes, we avoid eating fats because it makes us feel uncomfortable. If the liver is congested, it will affect the quality and viscosity of our blood, which adversely affects the blood vessel linings and the heart. Multiple pancreatic dysfunctions and pancreatic inflammation are connected to chronic liver or gallbladder congestion. Digestion of excessive or rancid fats and processed sugars can stress the liver, especially if it is already clogged with toxins from infections, harmful chemicals, and antibiotics.

Healthy fats that support our gut and are anti-inflammatory include whole food sources such as seeds (e.g., organic sesame seed oil and sunflower oil). Olive oil has many health-supporting properties and supports bile flow. Coconut oil has great immune supporting properties and aids thyroid function. It is important to include a variety of fats and oils. Fish contains omega-3 oils; however, choose only wild fish. (Mercury is a concern.)

Avoid all fried foods, sugary treats, excessive caffeine, and processed foods with harmful vegetable oils. Instead, eat healthy fats and a rainbow of vegetables that include phytonutrients, bioflavonoids, and carotenoids and add a naturally sweet, sour, and bitter taste to your daily menu.

Organic dark leafy vegetables, including dandelion, mustard greens, kale, spinach, chard, radishes, beets, and beet greens all support your liver. These are great whole food sources that target liver detox and bile flow. Bitter foods also help stimulate the bile flow, aiding digestion; this is one reason why Swedish bitters are very popular after a meal. Burdock, dandelion, licorice root (not with elevated blood pressure), or milk thistle tea after a meal can also enhance your digestion.

Cruciferous vegetables including cauliflower, cabbages, brussels sprouts, and broccoli support detox, add fiber to the diet, and protect against cancer.

Sulfur-rich whole food choices include garlic, ginger, and scallions. These also improve microcirculation to the eyes, fingers, feet, kidneys, and heart.

Steam or sauté dark leafy greens because they contain oxalic acid. Cooking neutralizes the oxalates; thus, the body is able to absorb the nutrients from the dark greens—calcium in particular. I am not a fan of the raw kale revolution because kale and other vegetables like broccoli must be exposed to low heat to neutralize certain inhibitors so that we can absorb all the nutrients of the plants.

Chlorophyll-rich foods include parsley, wheatgrass, spirulina, and cilantro; they support detoxification and the immune system. However, be aware that these are also high in oxalates, which can be a problem for some, especially if certain gut bacteria (oxalobacter species) that degraded the oxalates are insufficient. This is common in children who have been exposed to antibiotics at an early age.

Choline (or phosphatidylcholine) is very important for optimal gallbladder function. Choline is found in animal proteins, including eggs. It plays in important role in maintaining the integrity of our cell membranes, and it is needed for making neurotransmitters (brain chemicals). With chronic illness, we often need more than we can eat.

6. Beyond Food—What about Supplementation?

It is vital to get a large variety of nutrients into a tired and compromised body, especially as a jump start. This is why a whole food shake made with filtered water, mineral liquids, phytonutrients from green plants and berries, healthy oils, and spices can be very helpful. I recommend adding a protein powder, gelatin powder, goat yogurt, or, my favorite, raw egg yolks from healthy chickens that were raised on pasture to your shake. Be creative and choose foods that are in season where you live. It is simple to do, and it is nutrient-effective on many levels.

As a holistic practitioner, I believe in supplementation (to support biological function) with high-quality supplements to fast-track a gut-healing protocol. But supplementation must be assessed on an individual basis. Keep in mind that with persistent Lyme and antibiotic and other drug treatment, digestion, hormonal balance, and gut health are already compromised. What works for your partner or friend can have a totally different reaction in your body. *Only supplement once you have consulted with a qualified professional.*

Fillers, binders, synthetic colors, gluten, yeast, petroleum byproducts, and additional toxins (e.g., heavy metals) are concerns in nutritional supplements. Alcohol in herbal tinctures or homeopathic remedies can also be problematic for some individuals. All supplementation must be customized and carefully titrated because it all affects your unique biochemistry, inflammation, and immune tolerance. The sourcing of nutrients and ensuring the product is not contaminated with heavy metals or environmental pollutants are also important.

When the body is low on resilience, going back to nature and adding adaptogens or herbal tonics, such as rhodiola, ashwagandha, and rehmannia, will assist you in navigating the landscape of chronic Lyme or any treatment intervention. The brain and endocrine glands need additional support, and that must be part of any treatment protocol. (Check for contraindications with medications.) Herbal formulations are broad-spectrum in their healing powers because they influence the nervous, endocrine, and immune systems. Herbals work best in whole form and synergies, and a combination such as Siberian ginseng and licorice can provide powerful support with far-reaching effects. Nature has incredible wisdom, nutrition, and healing powers that we cannot synthesize in a lab—interestingly, nearly every pharmaceutical has a plant-based origin.

Supporting the gut lining and flora on a daily basis is imperative for individuals with chronic Lyme. I often recommend using additional supplementation to optimize digestion, with bitters and digestive enzymes and, in some cases, with hydrochloric acid. As I mentioned, products I use often include an oxbile and enzyme combo from Vital Nutrients, Biotics Research, Enzymedica, Gaia, Designs For Health, and Standard Process, but there are many options available.

A higher dose L-glutamine powder in a glass of water on an empty stomach (unless hyper-excitability, headaches, and glutamine sensitivity are already present), an herbal tea such as slippery elm or deglycyrrhized licorice, or a gut-healing complex of a variety of herbs, including marshmallow root, okra pepsin, slippery elm, or goldenseal, can provide gut lining support. Teas can be easy to combine with a meal; Mountain Rose Herbs produces some of my favorite teas. Berberine has antimicrobial, anti-inflammatory, and blood sugar balance supporting properties. (Please use caution with hypoglycemia and POTS.)

Zinc and vitamins A, C, D, K, and F are also in the mix for a healthy gut environment, lymph tissue, and mucosal lining—a rotation of nutritional and herbal products is very helpful on a long-term basis.

Gut flora support includes a wide and diverse spectrum. Major players are lactobacillus spp., bifidobacterium spp., and acidophilus. Probiotic choices can include Klaire Labs, Prescript Assists, VSL-3, or MegaSporeBiotic; I recommend rotating multiple strains. Diversity is what matters most.

A healthy yeast population in the gut can be bolstered with oral inoculation of a healthy yeast strain called *Saccharomyces boulardii*, which is also helpful with diarrhea. Colostrum and Lauricidin also contribute to gut mucosal integrity and immune modulation.

Liver and gallbladder support are part of every therapeutic program; you might consider supplementation with milk thistle because our toxic environment makes it challenging for our organs to detox efficiently.

Homemade vaginal suppositories made with coconut oil and *S. boulardii* or Mega Spore Biotics can be an option for a vaginal yeast infection, and an oral rinse made with *S. boulardii* or grapefruit seed extract can be helpful with thrush in the mouth. Oil pulling with coconut oil is another option. Essential oils have been helpful for many. Uva ursi, cranberry, D-mannose, goldenseal, green chiretta, and echinacea all support compromised immune functions that allow vaginal yeast infections to flourish.

A note of caution: Probiotics and healthy yeast can stir up the immune system and the harmful microbes. This can result in bloating, stomach pains, inflammation, a histamine response, and increased Lyme-related symptoms due to intolerance of specific strains or from the resulting die-off reaction of the bad bacteria or a herx reaction.

Nervous system fortification to improve the gut-brain connection can include Huperzine A, Neuroplex or Pituitrophin PMG from Standard Process, bacopa complex, CogniCare from Researched Nutritionals, inositol and vitamin B complex with activated vitamins (especially B6 and folate). There are many other choices.

Anti-inflammatories include boswellia, arnica, N-acetylcysteine (NAC), alpha-lipoic acid, high-quality omega-3 fatty acids in ratio with omega-6 fatty acids, evening primrose oil, cod liver oil, liposomal rhizols, vitamin D3 (cholecalciferol), Indian frankincense, liposomal turmeric, green tea extract, resveratrol, celery seed, and liposomal glutathione. Fiber supplementation might not be appropriate for everyone, and it can make gut symptoms worse if an overgrowth of harmful bacteria is present. It is contraindicated in some cases until the gut flora balance has improved.

Soluble fiber can include resistant starch, plantain flour, inulin, acacia, physillum husk, glucomannan powder, unmodified potato starch pectin, and guar gum. Physillum also assists in clearing elevated low-density lipoprotein cholesterol from the bloodstream. It is also helpful in blood sugar control, especially with elevated blood sugar. Be aware that fiber acts like a sweeper, and thus can *sweep out any medications or supplements you are using,* so take them an hour or two before eating high-fiber foods. Also make sure that you hydrate well; increasing your fiber intake when you are dehydrated can increase the risk of constipation. Choose what is appropriate for you.

Proteolytic enzymes (such as nattokinase, lumbrokinase, Interfase Plus, Wobenzyme products, and serrapeptase) can initiate a detox, since they are also involved in the breakdown of biofilms and infectious matter. However, they also have anti-inflammatory properties and support the cleanup of debris in the bloodstream. Enzymes also have blood-thinning properties that can be useful with increased blood viscosity and high fibrinogen associated with stealth infections. I use them in clinical practice with all chronic infections, including fungal infections, SIBO, scar tissue, and hemorrhoids.

When it comes to supplementation, I look for the less-chemical options if whole food supplements are not appropriate. If dairy is tolerated, a whole food, quality whey protein powder from Standard Process is supportive for the gut immune system and for detoxing harmful chemicals and poisons. For protein shakes, some tolerate a good pea protein, others with severe gastric troubles do better with a rice protein.

Any supplementation must be done with the guidance of a health-care professional because of possible interference with antibiotic treatment, psychiatric medications, blood pressure and blood sugar challenges, and individual sensitivities (even sensitivities to probiotic strains and histamine) come into play with a challenged gut.

. . . .

Wrapping Up

With Lyme-related infections, gut issues will be part of the picture. Do what you can, eat whole foods with optimal food preparation, hydrate well with electrolytes, and get enough rest.

As part of your Lyme journey, investigate and treat all underlying microbial challenges in the gut if you are not able to tolerate certain foods and suffer from abdominal pains. Toxins in commercial foods can mimic chronic Lyme symptoms, keeping you sick physically and psychologically because they place a strain on all organs and overwhelm detoxification pathways.

Do what you can and take it one day at a time. Make a big pot of broth so you always have some on hand, especially on days when you are not feeling well. Create a shopping list of foods you can tolerate, and add some gut-healing foods to your list.

Set some time aside to prepare food, and make a little extra so you have leftovers in the fridge or freezer. This will save you time and energy, but be sure to store them well to prevent spoilage or histamine buildup.

Before you get started, put on some classical music or something that you enjoy listening to—maybe even sing or hum along with the tune. The process of food preparation is creation in which you see, touch, hear, smell, and feel how you are part of a whole. The hardest thing is often having the time to do it, so decide which day is best for you and the time when you have more energy to shop, prepare, and cook. Nourish within and without in a peaceful environment.

"We need to listen to the patient's story and develop a response to it. The approach to complex syndromes may be much more profound than just trying to pound a round peg into a square hole to get a singular diagnosis."

—Dr. Jeffery Bland

Chapter Nine

What Goes In Must Go Out—
The Elimination Factor

We've spent a lot of time discussing the top of the digestive tube; let us now discuss what can happen at the bottom of the tube—in the bowels. We must consider the prior medical history of the individual before the Lyme and connected infections began. Were there challenges with constipation, food sensitivities, or digestive troubles before the Lyme-related infections? I include family history in this because in many cases, there are parents, aunts or uncles, or siblings who are experiencing digestive issues too—indicating a genetic predisposition. While addressing digestive and bowel challenges, it is best to pay attention to what foods make you feel well (or not) and the frequency, color, smell, and consistency of your stool. Be sure to write this down in a food diary for tracking purposes.

I hope that by now you have a much better understanding of how foods, medications, toxins, and gut infections can affect your ability to rebound toward wellness—and what you can do about it. I must reiterate though: Lyme and coinfections make everything much more complex. If multiple medications are in play, their side effects add to complications and nutrient deficiencies, besides being another toxic burden on an already compromised body. I know this can be completely overwhelming, especially as many physicians neither accept nor know about the impact of Lyme, SIBO, food sensitivities, and nutrient deficiencies.

Constipation and diarrhea are common, and both bring additional challenges into the Lyme infection scenario. It must also be considered that the Lyme infection is the root cause of these challenges, and therapeutic interventions must be made accordingly. Changing symptoms and disabling fatigue can also occur when antimicrobial cycling, antibiotic treatment, and therapeutic detox strategies are implemented, resulting in constipation and diarrhea. Antibiotic-associated diarrhea is another concern.

The liver and gallbladder drain into the small intestine; with thickened bile, the inner filtration system does not work well and toxins spill back out into the blood stream, irritating and inflaming the immune system. Gallbladder stones can form, as well as kidney stones, and both can create pain and inflammation, with slowed transit time in the bowels. This will cause more symptoms of ill health, too.

Any blockage in the elimination pathways will create undesirable reactions. This can affect skin health, sleep, grinding of teeth, moods, bloating, increased urination during the night, psychiatric symptoms, lower back pain, headaches, swelling in the legs and ankles, carbohydrate cravings, neck and shoulder pain, weight gain, and brain fog. Diarrhea creates other symptoms including cramping, mineral deficiencies, and dehydration. Chronic constipation might result in a visit to the emergency room to remove impacted waste. It is of utmost importance to address all of the possible root causes that contribute to these problems.

Certain nutrients, such as magnesium citrate, high doses of vitamin C, or fiber, optimal hydration, enemas or colonics, avoidance of iced or cold drinks and foods, and prune juice can be helpful for symptomatic relief of constipation.

Gently nudge the body and remind it of its ability to function and flow, because with nutrient depletion and infections, it will hit speed bumps along the way. Where and when depends on the individual. Imagine that the detoxification and elimination process is like a car. All parts must function properly so the car can be driven. There is no point in having a car with a great engine and a new steering wheel if the car has no tires or no gas in the tank or the exhaust tube is blocked. It is the same with detoxification in the liver and other elimination channels in the body.

Of course, heavy metal detoxification sounds like a great idea; however, how compromised are the various biological systems in the body, and how much energy is available to support a heavy metal detox? Is the body low in minerals? These are questions that must be asked. With a metal detox, it is possible to drive the metals deeper into the tissues where they create more health problems. It should never be the starting point when dealing with vector-borne infections. Instead, it is much better to start with a gentle detox by eating a variety of whole foods that provide many of the nutrients required for gentle detoxification and glutathione production. Heavy metal detoxification is often essential at a later stage in treatment with these persistent infections, but this must be done under the supervision of a professional.

To neutralize toxins, the body needs targeted therapies to support production of glutathione. This antioxidant is often low in individuals whose systems are compromised, and use of vitamins C and E, lipoic acid, N-acetyl cysteine, methylfolate, glycine, B12, S-Adenosyl methionine, pyridoxal phosphate, magnesium, zinc, selenium, and others can all be supportive detox agents. Please understand that this is not a supplement prescription; it gives you a comprehensive glimpse into the complexities of detoxification at a cellular level. It is important to nudge and nourish the body and not to overwhelm it with super-dose pill or tablet supplementation, especially if you are having detox, genetic variables, and digestive troubles already.

Our stool provides us with information regarding what is occurring in the gut ecology, the gallbladder, and the colon; yet, when it comes to the digestive system and microbial immune system, there is a lot we still do not know. Many species cannot be studied because they cannot be cultured outside the host, and everyone has a different microbial community in their gut. Bowel function also mirrors our stress and our emotions.

A healthy colon contains a densely populated and diverse ecosystem. If you live in the United Stated and travel to Japan for a vacation, the local foods there will alter your microbiome. However, upon your return home, the microbiome will rebalance itself to its prior ecology. This is also why diarrhea is common when drinking unfiltered water in foreign countries. The locals there can drink tap water because their gut microbes have adapted to the microbes in their tap water.

Long-term diets that exclude various food groups will also cause an alteration in the microbial balance, and that too can contribute to health challenges in the colon. Butyrate production is severely compromised in many individuals, especially with prolonged antibiotic use that affects the diversity of the micro-flora. A gluten-free diet will decrease the health-supporting bifidia strains even more. We need these for the production of butyrate. A healthy bowel movement should be easy to pass in an "elegant swoosh." It should smell and look like healthy soil in the ground, and it should sink to the bottom of the bowl. The regularity, color, shape, consistency, and whether the stool sinks or floats are all important factors. Is there a film on the water like a thin layer of grease, or is the stool runny, or yellowish and difficult to pass? Just as it is important to see what goes into the body, it is also important to observe what comes out of the body (or not), especially with the challenges of chronic Lyme.

Any therapeutic antibiotic, intravenous glutathione treatment, or herbal intervention can result in a severe backlash if constipation is in play. With con-stipation, the body reabsorbs the toxins into the blood stream, and this can make you very ill, as well as affect your mood and ability to think clearly. The toxic overload adds severe stress on the kidneys and the liver, as both are filtration systems. The auto-intoxication also creates additional inflammation in the body, sometimes creating severe symptoms that require hospitalization.

Stagnant matter and toxins in the bowels become a feeding ground for opportunistic microbes, such as yeast, parasites, and bacteria. Often, antifungal medications such as nystatin or fluconazole are prescribed for yeast overgrowth during antibiotic treatment for persistent Lyme. But these infections can be tenacious; chronic and persistent Lyme infections suppress the immune system, allowing opportunistic fungal infections in the intestines and colon to prolifer-ate. It is important to support the terrain of the gut immune system during any Lyme treatment and after treatment has discontinued.

Symptoms of constipation include abdominal bloating, back pain, head-aches, stools that are hard to pass, mucous production, gassiness, anal fis-sures, and increased risk of hemorrhoids, even ruptured hemorrhoids. If bowel movements are too frequent, you could end up with severe dehydration, malnutrition, unwanted weight loss, and low blood pressure, making you feel faint, dizzy, and weak.

For additional information regarding challenges with elimination, a test for

SIBO or a four-day comprehensive digestive stool analysis home test from a specialized lab can be helpful. But keep in mind that these tests can be negative despite clinical findings. There are many variables that can interfere with stool test results, including self-destruction of microbes, moon cycles, cyst forms, interference from residual medications, and herbal supplementation; there are also financial considerations when it comes to advanced testing.

Additional challenges that can contribute to bowel dysfunctions include a lack of fiber in the diet, heavy metal toxicity, poorly controlled diabetes, a hypothyroid condition, lactose intolerance, celiac disease, aging, and structural abnormalities of the gut and biofilm.[1] Studies are constantly being updated, yet it is well documented that acid-blocking and antibiotic medications can play an important role in causing or contributing to SIBO, SIFO, and chronic intestinal transit challenges.

With elimination challenges, it is imperative to consider the many possible root causes:

- Thyroid dysfunction
- Use of antacids with calcium carbonate
- Iron pills
- Lactose intolerance
- Gallbladder and liver congestion
- Hormonal fluctuations
- Infections in the gut, including *H-pylon*, parasites, bacteria, and fungal overgrowth
- Stress
- Prior food poisoning
- Gluten intolerance
- Dehydration
- Inactivity
- Excessive coffee, caffeine, or sugar consumption
- Brain inflammation
- Lack of fiber in the diet
- Food sensitivities
- Travel

- Lack of hydrochloric acid and pancreatic enzymes
- Histamine intolerance, salicylate sensitivity
- Hemorrhoids

Supporting the Gut-Brain Axis

Homeopathy with *Sarcodes*, Emotional Freedom Technique (EFT), acupuncture, and energy medicine are alternative healing options for reactivation of damaged nerves that can be used to restore nerve function in the bowels.

One highly recommended extract is huperzine A; its dosage must be customized until a therapeutic effect is achieved. Other supplements that positively affect the gut and brain chemicals (including serotonin and dopamine) include acetylcholine, 5-hydroxytryptophan, phosphatidylcholine, and L-tyrosine. Tangerine peel is creating renewed interest.

If you have had no success with various dietary and digestive interventions mentioned in previous chapters, consider these options. This is cutting-edge information not typically addressed in commercial medicine.

According to Dr. Datis Kharrazian, the vagus nerve response, which also fires into the brain, is activated in all the modalities discussed in this section. This reconnects communication between the gut-brain axis, which has become dysfunctional as a result of infections, brain trauma and inflammation, and a leaky gut. Investigate which of these is best for you, especially if you have a history of chronic constipation and have already tried various remedies without success.

Try gargling vigorously for a few minutes a few times a day, until the tears come, to increase the vagal nerve connection, which controls and activates the palate muscles in the back of the throat. If the muscle tone is weak, it can be difficult to gargle vigorously. It is best to start with a small amount of water by the sink, so you can spit it out quickly if you feel uncomfortable. To make it a routine practice, consider gargling each time you go to the bathroom. It must be done frequently, because this action is about muscle conditioning.

Singing out loud activates brain fibers and reestablishes the connection of the gut and the brain. It might be easier to sing along to a song on the radio or your phone. Again, this must be done a few times day, for a few minutes each time, to improve and condition the muscles.

Another option is to buy a box of tongue scrapers and use them to provoke the gag reflex, by pushing down on the back of the tongue. You can feel your eyes tear up as you activate the muscles in the palate that are fired by the vagus nerve. This method is helpful in activating the gut-brain reflex and should be done a few times a day.

An organic coffee enema done at home is another option. The caffeine engages the liver and gallbladder. Caffeine promotes bile flow and stimulates peristalsis; after a little time, you will feel the urge to eliminate (accidents do happen). To retrain the gut-brain nervous system connection, suppress the urge to eliminate. If there is no urge to eliminate, it means that more caffeine will be required to stimulate peristalsis. Go slow; it takes practice, and the coffee concentration depends on what you can handle. (Some individuals cannot tolerate coffee.) Increasing retention duration and concentration of the coffee has a training effect on the gut-brain axis.

The bottom line is that the gut and brain must communicate with each other in order to restore flow in the digestive tract. Food eliminations upstream are essential and infections and immune weaknesses in the gastric tube must be dealt with. For challenges with elimination, it is important not to only focus on the problem area in the bowels but also on the problems upstream, because that is usually where you can often find additional root causes.

. . . .

Wrapping Up

There is a psychological and emotional connection when it comes to bodily functions. An imbalance between the rational mind and our emotions stresses our digestive system and can manifest in any number of symptoms.

If you feel uptight, angry, and tense, perhaps worried that you might lose your job or cannot afford treatment, or you are frustrated by the long-term and repeated misdiagnosis of your Lyme illness, or you feel misunderstood by those around you, the liver, intestines, and colon will be affected.

An emotional paralysis in daily life will be mirrored in elimination challenges in the bowels. Constipation can also be connected to the stress of holding on to something or being a perfectionist. These emotions instill images of tightness, congestion, and tension, and this is reflected in the body. If you feel anxious and jittery, so does the colon. In either case, mind-body calming techniques and biofeedback techniques can be very helpful in optimizing bowel activity. It is at this level that we can make healing interventions that allow our body renewed well-being and energy.

"The digestive canal represents a tube passing through the entire organism and communicating with the external world, i.e. as it were the external surface of the body, but turned inwards and thus hidden in the organism."

—IVAN PAVLOV

Chapter Ten

Action Steps For Constipation and Diarrhea Resolution

With chronic constipation, over-the-counter or herbal laxatives are commonly used as a desperate measure to get the bowels to move. Initially, they might be successful; however, overuse of laxatives will impede your natural transit ability and weaken the bowel muscles, making things worse for you in the long term. The goal is to restore bowel function instead of enabling lifetime dependency on laxatives for symptom relief.

I. Creating an Optimal Eating Environment

Put on some music, take some deep breaths, anoint yourself with some calming essential oils, or light a candle—take time to reduce your stress. You want to shift from the fight-or-flight response into the calming response of the parasympathetic nervous system. This is foundational in initiating optimal digestion from the top of the digestive loop.

Create a peaceful, nourishing environment by sitting down when eating and not eating on the go. Drinking a teaspoon of raw apple cider vinegar in a glass of water before a meal optimizes the pH (supporting protein digestion). Become mindful of and grateful for the foods nature provides. Good food preparation and chewing until the food becomes a liquid in your mouth will activate the digestive process, starting in the brain, nose, and mouth.

Ensure optimal hydration with clean water *between* meals, but avoid drinking water *during* meals. You do not want to dilute your stomach acid.

Tight and restrictive clothing also impedes digestion, especially when sitting for a long period of time. Think about how those clothes create stagnation in your blood and lymphatic flow. Change into comfortable clothes, so that your body can flow and digestive organs are at ease. If possible, take off your shoes, and place your feet on the floor. Get connected to the grounding power of the earth.

Turn the TV and other technological devices off and come back into your present and calm environment. The electromagnetic frequencies (EMF) of technological devices affect enzymes, hormones in our bodies, and electric functions in our brain, decreasing our digestive capacity. Plus, we are mentally distracted and not fully paying attention to what, or how much, we are eating. In this scenario, it is easy to overeat because the gut and brain are disconnected.

2. Healthy Hydration and Whole Food Options That Support Transit

Adequate hydration is the first step in healthy elimination function. If you are dehydrated, water will be removed from the waste material to be reused in the body; the waste in the transit tube can increase in thickness or turn into stones that are hard to pass. You can start your day by drinking lemon juice or raw apple cider vinegar in a glass of water to gently nudge elimination and detox. Add a touch of sea salt—this increases absorption of water by the cells and replenishes electrolytes.

Are you hydrating but running to the restroom soon after? Despite drinking a lot of water, are you still thirsty and feel the need to drink more? This is a sign that you are not absorbing water into your cells. Instead, it is going right through your body. The adrenals are involved in this scenario too; they play an important role in the fluid balance (and blood pressure). Excessive urination will increase electrolyte depletion, making you even more thirsty and dehydrated in your body's tissues. Lack of electrolytes, such as sodium and potassium, stresses the kidneys. The addition of electrolytes, Celtic sea salt, or Himalayan salt with a little lemon, lime, or freshly squeezed orange juice in a glass of water is an option. Stevia or a little raw honey can also be added—stir it up into a refreshing mix. A little watermelon juice or raw coconut water and fresh herbs such as mint, rosemary, or nettles are tasty inclusions on a hot summer day. (Be aware of the overall sugar content, especially with coconut water or fruit juices.)

Lyme and coinfections can be embedded in the urogenital tract, bladder, or prostate, causing great inflammation, pain, and frequent but incomplete voiding. Adrenal fatigue, a toxic liver, a urinary tract infection or cystitis, an inflamed bladder or prostate, or a lack of minerals can contribute to excessive voiding during the day as well as frequent urination during the night.

Drinking a warm glass of water in the morning on an empty stomach can promote the gastric-colonic reflex in the large intestine to ease constipation. For some individuals, a cup of coffee provides the elimination stimulus because it irritates the bowels. During the day, consumption of warm water will support normal spasmodic bowel activity if antispasmodic teas (such as chamomile, peppermint, ginger, fennel, or anise tea) are not available.

Elimination-supporting foods, including homemade lassi, yogurt, or kefir, can be a helpful option for some. (Coconut milk kefir or yogurt can be an option for those who cannot tolerate dairy.) Fermented foods such as sauerkraut or fermented carrots provide whole food probiotics and a predigested source of fiber that, if tolerated, support gut flora and elimination.

For some individuals, raw cabbage juice or prune juice can be helpful to ease constipation; however, the sugar content in prune juice will feed any fungal or microbial infection and can disrupt blood sugar balance.

THE ROLE OF FIBER: HERE IT IS AGAIN . . .

Soluble fiber (oatmeal, blueberries, beans, apples, prunes, figs) absorbs water and becomes a gel-like mush; it slows transit, and makes stools softer and easier to pass.

Insoluble fiber is the strong, sinewy fiber in foods like celery, plantains, inulin in chicory, and bananas. Vegetables are a good source of fiber; however, they can be fermented internally and create bloating and gas if the microflora in the gut is out of balance. Fiber-rich vegetables can contribute to constipation, including irritable bowel syndrome (IBS), small intestinal bacterial overgrowth (SIBO), and yeast overgrowth.

Fiber can either help or compound symptoms connected with constipation or diarrhea, yet we require adequate fiber in our diet to support the production of butyrate (short-chain fatty acids) that are also prebiotics. If you are on a grain-free diet plan, supplementation of fiber is warranted; you might not be getting sufficient fiber in your daily foods to support prebiotics, stool formation, and optimal transit in the bowels. Fiber plays in important role in sweeping out of accumulated toxic waste, especially with antibiotic treatment.

Another way to increase your daily fiber intake is by adding two tablespoons of freshly ground flaxseeds into your shake, oatmeal, or over your vegetables. It is best to keep organic flaxseeds in the fridge and grind them right before you sprinkle them on your food. (Avoid the prepackaged ground flaxseeds that are already rancid.) A combination of chia seeds, sunflower seeds, and flaxseed is also an option, especially if you are on a grain-free or temporary low FODMAP diet plan. Soak these seeds overnight to increase digestibility and bioavailability of nutrients.

It is essential to maintain optimal hydration with additional fiber; otherwise, symptoms associated with constipation and bloating in the abdominal area can worsen. If you supplement with fiber or seeds, start slow and allow the body to process the increased fiber. Not doing so can result in gas, bloating, and constipation. It can take up to three days for the gut to regulate itself; however, if symptoms persist, it warrants further investigation.

Since the nervous system is implicated in chronic constipation, integrating whole foods (e.g., cod liver oil) that nourish the brain and nerves is helpful.

A lack of fat and healthy oil in the diet can be a component in constipation, too. These provide lubrication and aid in stool formation. Omega-3 and omega-6 fatty acids are found most abundantly in free-range animal and plant sources. Small wild-sourced fish, such as sardines, also contain healthy oils, which have anti-inflammatory properties. Coconut oil, if tolerated, provides energy to an inflamed brain and a tired thyroid, which are involved in intestinal motility, or peristalsis. The addition of bile salts (as well as enzymes and hydrochloric acid) might alleviate symptoms of constipation, but this option must first be discussed with a professional.

3. Regular Exercise to Increase Visceral Circulation and Lymphatic Drainage

Muscular contractions, with gentle and repetitive pumping movements, increase circulation and respiration of the internal organs. Blood flow to the intestines is essential to facilitate elimination, and muscle activity is required to promote removal of toxins from the cells, lymphatic drainage, and nourishment with oxygen.

Moderate bouncing or rebounding movements and repetitive squatting motions can induce peristalsis with the increase of overall circulation. If ten to fifteen minutes is tolerated, this will be helpful in encouraging lymphatic detox and mental wellness. Gentle use of an elliptical trainer or a rebounder can be supportive in releasing stagnation within elimination pathways. The goal is to promote blood flow and to build energy with improved circulation, with the added benefit of reducing mental stress, anxiety, and depression. Make sure not to overdo it; you will be wiped out for the rest of the day if you do. Constipation is associated with stagnation; if the body is moving, the bowels are more likely to move.

Gentle squatting movements increase blood flow in the intestines and help stimulate bowel activity and motility. As oxygen is brought to the cells, muscle tension and constriction in the bowels lessens and gas buildup decreases. Squatting and rhythmic motions with deep breaths have a massaging effect on the colon and increases the tone of the intra-abdominal muscles, organs, and pelvic floor. This will assist in decreasing stagnation in the colon; however, painful knee and hip joints must be taken into consideration with squats. (Other options that follow might be more appropriate for you.)

Swimming can be a great way to ease tightness and maintain flexibility of painful joints. It aids in circulation without stressing inflamed joints. Exercise in the water is especially helpful when Lyme-related vertigo makes balance very challenging. Use of a buoyancy belt can be helpful for treading water in the pool, as will pool noodles and floats. (The toxic chlorine in public swimming pools is a deterrent for many. Also, indoor pool areas are often moist and humid, creating other mold, sinus, and respiratory health-related challenges.)

Working up a mild sweat is helpful because the skin also serves as an organ of elimination. Some have no tolerance to movement, which results in increased body temperature. Hard-core and fatigue-inducing exercise are best avoided. Cardio training or endurance training is contraindicated; exercising with a prolonged elevated heart rate strains the heart and adrenals and lowers immune function, which are already compromised. (And you will feel even more wiped out.) At times, taking care of household chores is exercise enough, or even too much, if you are going through a tough time.

When it comes to exercise, weight training is helpful, but you must be careful; less is more. Strength training will support growth hormones, improve function, and build needed muscle and bone. If weight loss is desired, short interval weight training will support insulin sensitivity and metabolic function. Use of machines in a gym can be helpful to increase muscle tone and functional strength; however, use extreme caution, because antibiotics and malnourishment can weaken tendons. The use of Swiss balls and gentle core training can decrease joint pain and improve joint stability and mood. Listen to your body. The body needs movement and flow on a daily basis to clear toxins within the lymphatic system and to restore resilience, but do not push it too hard—you will increase fatigue and pain if you overdo it. It is best to have an initial meeting with a fitness professional who understands your goals, pain, and energy challenges.

A daily stretching program with fluid and repetitive movements helps to remove waste and toxins out of cells. You can do this at home in a controlled environment, especially if you are heat sensitive. Rhythmic stretching helps to maintain flexibility in tight muscles and supports circulation and oxygenation of the cells in the body. It also dials down an overactive brain, emotional stress, and a cramping colon. This gentle, therapeutic approach is a stress-reducing modality, reducing the fight-or-flight response.

Of course fatigue, nerve pain, and joint pain must be considered in any exercise or movement program. Gentle massage and yoga are both helpful in restoring the lymphatic and circulatory systems. They do not demand high amounts of energy and can provide movement and stress reduction when you are exhausted and in pain. If you enjoy dancing, go ahead and sing along too; it will encourage more energy and healing as you bring joy, music, and laughter into your life. Qigong is also very energy-building and gentle, with movements that assist organ and glandular function. Easy walks in nature are restorative, and they improve circulation and promote bowel activity. Choose any movement modality that resonates with you: Move regularly, and be sure to rest afterward.

4. Breathing Exercises to Promote Flow and Stress Reduction

This stress-reducing self-help modality eases the irritated and constipated digestive tract and colon. Take in a deep breath through the nose. Focus on expanding the diaphragm and abdominal area when you inhale, instead of just using your chest, shoulders, and neck. Pause. Then exhale through the mouth, fully integrating the abdominal area. Pause. Practice this in front of a mirror, and take note of how you breathe. Each pause is like a full stop at the end of a sentence. Over time, slow down and steady the rhythm: just like the waves of the ocean, rolling back and forth on the beach. Establish a slow rhythm that works for you. If you place your hands on the abdominal area, you can reconnect to the source of life, your breath. You can feel it. Do what you can. If it works for you, that is great. (If it makes you anxious, discontinue, and consider another stress reducing modality.)

By becoming mindful of how we breathe and with what intention, we can calm down the gut and brain. This practice integrates the lungs and digestive tone, and it reduces stress. With Lyme and coinfections, the body is more on edge in chronic fight-or-flight mode; thus, more attention must be given to stress reduction modalities, including meditation, breaks during the day, listening to classical music, gardening, preparing a home-cooked meal, watching the flames in a fireplace or of a burning candle, and breathing exercises. Find a way to integrate sacred time into your daily life, even if just for a few minutes. Breathing consciously is something you have the power to do; you can do it anywhere, and it does not cost anything.

Emotional Freedom Technique (EFT) is a form of psychological acupressure that uses a tapping motion on various parts of the body. If this resonates with you, take time during the day to practice and allow yourself to rebalance on an energetic level. Find a comfortable place and take off your glasses, jewelry, and wristwatch, and place any technological devices as far away from your body as possible. Use affirmations that are specific to your needs as you allow yourself this special time to enhance your ability to live with the challenges of your daily life.

5. A Mechanical Perspective

It is important to note that our modern-day toilet does not support bowel elimination. Traditional squatting during elimination (in a position where your thighs are brought up closer toward your torso) is very helpful with chronic elimination problems.

The traditional, primal squatting position changes the spatial relationships of the intestinal organs and musculature, relaxing and straightening the rectum. By placing the feet on a footstool, you can recreate this optimal position that supports the mechanics in a constipated elimination pathway.

The development of the Western toilet has created a disadvantage for our colon. Toilet stools that curve around the bottom of your toilet or a small step stool can help to ease your painful elimination challenges.

6. Supplementation: Need Green Medicine Relief?

We must look upstream in the digestive tract when dealing with chronic constipation. Supplements for brain support include choline, huperzine, and protomorphogens from Standard Process. Herbal and homeopathic adaptogens including rhodiola, rehmannia, German chamomile, and licorice will stimulate digestive function. Stress affects our brain and, in turn, our digestive tract. It is important to consider a whole body approach when dealing with chronic Lyme.

Always chew your food well. Digestive enzymes, bitters, including gentian and wormwood, fruit peel or tangerine, hydrochloric acid (caution with gastritis or symptoms of *H. pylori*), and ox bile extract are helpful for many with ongoing constipation and gas. Standard Process, MediHerb, Biotics Research, Thorne, Designs For Health, Gaia, Allergy Research, Enzymedica, and Vital Nutrients are just a few companies that make digestive aids.

Magnesium citrate and magnesium oxide, higher-dose vitamin C (ascorbic acid), and triphala dissolved overnight in water are helpful in assisting bowel motility. These are to be considered temporary measures only; they provide symptom relief but can create dependence and do not restore natural function. When there is constipation associated with Lyme, medications, and SIBO, it is sometimes essential to use green medicine for a prolonged period of time because infections wreak havoc in the digestive system.

Bile salts, teas such as chanca piedra, or raw apple cider vinegar with lemon in water all help dissolve gallstones and thin the bile. (Chanca piedra also breaks up kidney stones and oxalates in the joints.) Dandelion, burdock, essiac, or milk thistle teas shore up liver function; it is best to buy loose-leaf. The addition of goldenseal and slippery elm will also assist the flow of waste and mucosal lining in the tract.

There are many probiotic options for enhancing gut flora balance. Eliminate products that contain FOS (fructooligosaccharide), GOS (galacto-oligosaccharide), MOS (mannan oligosaccharide), arabinogalactan, and inulin with constipation concerns, and rule out underlying microbial overgrowth. Avoid fiber supplementation if SIBO and microbial infections are in play. In infants, the strains *Lactobacillus reuteri*, *Lactobacillus casei*, and *Bifidobacterium breve* are helpful with relieving constipation (and colic). In adults, soil-based organisms such as PrescriptAssist, spores like MegaSpore, and probiotics containing *Saccharomyces boulardii*, *L. plantarum*, *Lactobacillus rhamnosus*, and *Bifidobacterium lactis* may be useful. Prokinectics that promote intestinal motility are helpful for many, especially for those with slowed transit time.

The above supplement suggestions are for general information purposes *only*. Consult with a professional before any supplementation as your needs are unique.

7. Complementary Treatments

Liver congestion, nerve damage in the transit pathways, insufficient digestion, and pituitary dysfunction are all implicated when it comes to severe bowel congestion. Additional modalities that address chronic constipation can include chiropractic care, homeopathy, energy medicine, ozone therapy, infrared saunas, acupuncture, visceral massage, and the Rife machine.

A gentle abdominal massage of the internal organs will also ease a constipated bowel. Choose essential oils that resonate with you and be gentle; an inflamed gut cannot take a lot of pressure. The massage can also stir up toxins. Before the massage, hydrate well with a warm glass of water with raw apple cider vinegar to help flush out toxins while provoking sluggish bowel activity. On You-Tube there are some great self-massage tutorials. Choose one that appeals to you and make that part of your routine for stress reduction and rest, while supporting your detox and elimination. Again, this is something you can do when you have quiet time. Create a comfortable and relaxing environment and reconnect with your body.

Chiropractic care and craniosacral care improve organ function and should be considered as well. Top sports medicine doctor and chiropractor Dr. Scott Duke, of Duke Chiropractic in New York City, asserts that treating underlying imbalances in the spine will affect the parasympathetic nerves in the sacrum, which are associated with elimination challenges. Yet, adjustments can also initiate a Lyme flare as spirokeets hide in joints. Keep this in mind when living with Lyme disease.

Toxicity is a contributing cause of chronic disease, yet this is neither addressed nor accepted in commercial medicine. Enemas, as mentioned earlier, are very helpful in assisting with detoxification and chronic constipation. Many people think of enemas as way-out procedures. They are not. Until the 1970s they were considered commercial treatments, as outlined in the Merck Manual that was used as a primary reference book by physicians. Today, they are viewed as a form of alternative medicine, and instead there is a great emphasis on pharmaceutical treatments and symptom suppression with no consideration of the concept for the need to detox with any chronic illness.

The are various enema options in a conventional setting. A common one is the saline enema available at drug stores. This is used to cleanse the bowels before a medical rectal examination and colonoscopy. A barium enema is used for a contrast x-ray to check for pathology in the small and large intestine.

The cleansing enema is very helpful to get rid of accumulated toxins and debris when using a binding agent such as bentonite clay or activated charcoal that can induce constipation. It is retained for a short period only and stimulates peristalsis that culminates in a bowel movement, often providing instant relief. Symptoms of bloating and gas indicate toxic waste, and with Lyme infections it is important to get rid of waste on a regular basis—especially if constipation is present.

Retention enemas, held for about fifteen minutes, stimulate the liver and gallbladder and encourage the release of toxic bile. This decreases the risk of autointoxication associated with constipation, endotoxins, herx reactions with Lyme treatment, gut infections, and a lack of intestinal motility. Coffee is often used in alternative cancer therapies as coffee stimulates the bile flow. (Avoid coffee enemas with palpitations, heart symptoms, hypogylcemia, POTS, anxiety, insomnia, kidney problems, and if you do not tolerate coffee.) Other options are raw apple cider vinegar, chlorophyll, burdock root, and butyrate (break open capsules).

Enemas can induce electrolyte imbalances when coffee is used. It is also important to recolonize and remineralize the colon because minerals and health-supporting flora also get washed out with the toxins during the enema. There are many informative resources available online that can guide you through the DIY enema process, but be sure and discuss this with a professional first. If you do not feel comfortable doing this at home, seek out a European-type wellness center or a colonic specialist.

Rectal ozonated antimicrobials, probiotics suppositories, or probiotic butyrate enemas are powerful and direct delivery options. These are very helpful if there are serious digestive troubles that limit digestibility and absorption of oral supplements. As fecal transplants are gaining acceptance for their success with *C. difficile* infections, there is a renewed interest in enemas. Yet many prefer to only drink their coffee, which does not have the therapeutic effects of a coffee enema.

Ozone therapy is widely accepted in Europe as a detoxification, anti-inflammatory, and immune-boosting modality. It has many applications in cancers and autoimmune diseases, including chronic colitis and chronic hepatitis. Rectal ozone treatments to stimulate liver and cellular detoxification are minimally invasive and done by a medical professional, unless one has a machine at home. The membranes of the small intestine directly absorb the ozone molecules, which enter the blood and then the liver. All the blood that passes through the liver comes in contact with the ozone. Toxins are removed, inflammation is reduced, and the cells vitality is increased.

Castor oil packs are a simple and inexpensive favorite, and they provide great therapeutic value. With liver and gallbladder challenges, the castor oil pack is something you can integrate into your self-care. The good news is that after the initial investment, it will pay for itself in the long term. The great news is that it does not involve swallowing another pill. Castor oil comes from the castor seed, and it is used for its lymph-stimulating and liver-detoxing properties, especially if used on the right side of the body. These were highly recommended by psychic healer Edgar Cayce as part of his healing protocols for constipation, pain, inflammation, uterine fibroids, and more.

Castor oil packs can be messy, and it stains, so you want to wear old clothes and use an old sheet. Castor oil packs are very effective, and they also allow you to have some needed quiet time during the process. This procedure requires high-quality (hexane free) castor oil on cotton flannel (which can be reused), a wraparound pack (plastic wrap is not optimal, but can be used), and a hot water bottle or heating pad that is placed on the pack. There are castor oil pack kits available from Radiant Life and other sellers online.

These action steps are helpful with chronic constipation, especially when you are in the midst of a specific Lyme antibiotic or detox treatment (for example, intravenous glutathione) or you are cycling a drug or herbal therapy and are experiencing constipation and chronic pain challenges. Consult with a professional before adding any treatment or supplement to your program. There are many options, so choose what feels right for you under the supervision of a trained professional only.

Excessive Elimination: Top Five Self-Help Actions

Too-frequent elimination or chronic diarrhea can manifest as increased urgency, elimination within an hour of eating, loose and runny stools, or exceeding three eliminations a day. These issues affect your quality of life—you can become afraid to leave the house. This is debilitating on so many levels. It can cause dehydration, malnourishment, depression, hopelessness, and relationship troubles; you might not be able to go to work or might not want to travel anymore. All possible root causes must be investigated. Food sensitivities and hidden infections must be investigated; yet other triggers, including histamine, salicylate sensitivity, and anxiety, can also cause hyperactivity of the colon. Lyme-related infections and antibiotics are an additional challenge in this inflammatory labyrinth. Excessive elimination, too, is of great concern: Cramping, heart palpitations, chronic fatigue, low blood pressure, fear of leaving the home, extreme weight loss, and muscle wasting are part of this challenging and energy-draining scenario. When transit time is too short, there is reduced nutrient absorption, which results in malnourishment and dehydration with loss of electrolytes. All affect blood sugar balance, stamina, hormones, concentration, blood pressure, and mood. You will feel drained and tired.

A lack of vitamin B12 is of concern in this scenario because a deficiency can create issues that could mimic Lyme-related symptoms. These include palpitations, nerve disorders, or pain as well as memory and mood disorders. Vitamin B12 injections are helpful for many; discuss this with your physician (sublingual drops or tablets may also be an option). You should also monitor vitamin D levels with your doctor.

Chronic diarrhea can also be related to gallbladder dysfunction, and it can be a side effect after gallbladder removal. The addition of binders and bile salts can be very helpful, and dietary modifications may be required (a low-fat diet). These are all additional complications that must be taken into account in the overall picture of too-frequent elimination.

Excess production of histamine can also contribute to diarrhea and too-frequent elimination. Inflammation is also involved in the process, and histamine and salicylate factors must be kept in mind when dietary recommendations are made. Some common high-histamine foods include cheese (especially if aged), eggplant, mushrooms, yeast breads, sour cream, and fermented foods such as sauerkraut, soy sauce, coleslaw, pickles, mayo, and chili sauce. For salicylates foods, see chapter twelve. Genetic factors, enzyme dysfunction, and gut flora imbalances all are contributing players with histamine and salicylate accumulation.

I. SUBCLINICAL OPPORTUNISTIC AND HIDDEN STEALTH INFECTIONS

Too-frequent elimination challenges can be connected to prior unresolved food poisonings, chronic respiratory ailments, gut flora imbalances, breaches in the intestinal gut mucosa (leaky gut), opportunistic infections, and chronic inflammation that can drive autoimmune diseases in the bowels. An intolerance of medications, including antibiotics used in Lyme treatment, must be considered in every case as a causal or contributing factor.

A check must be done for *C. difficile* infection when chronic diarrhea is present, especially after or during antibiotic treatment. In severe cases, fast-acting pharmaceutical agents, including steroids, are necessary for acute crisis management while the root causes are investigated.

Ask your physician if herbal or homeopathic alternatives are not an option. With a challenged immune system and suboptimal detox system, medications like oral antibiotics, antacids, and steroids open the door for fungal and viral infections, digestive irritation, dysbiosis (including SIBO), nausea, fibromyalgia, chronic fatigue syndrome, and more. These also hamper your resilience. Educate yourself on the side effects when taking medications besides antibiotics; you can mitigate some of them with nutrients including CoQ10, alpha lipoc acid, fatty acids, and L-glutamine, probiotics, herbal teas, gut lining support, homeopathic remedies, and botanicals.

2. AUTOIMMUNE DIAGNOSIS? FOOD SENSITIVITIES ALWAYS COME INTO PLAY

Gluten intolerance and celiac disease must be ruled out with chronic diarrhea. An elimination diet is best, yet cross contamination from other foods can occur. Genetic testing can be helpful to uncover certain predispositions that can open the door for gluten, dairy, and histamine intolerance. However, it is important not to get too hung up on one factor when it comes to digestive disease management.

Additional functional testing is helpful; however, tests are not one hundred percent foolproof. Plus, they are not affordable for many who are already strained with the financial implications of Lyme-related treatment, long-term medications, and inability to work.

With ongoing diarrhea, food sensitivities must also be considered. Start with targeted therapeutic elimination of gluten, grains, dairy, eggs, citrus, corn, soy, nuts, nightshades, high FODMAP foods, and foods high in histamine and oxalates (salicylate sensitivity must also be considered). If symptoms improve, give the body time to settle down after being irritated and severely inflamed. Rebuild immune tolerance and gut flora balance by avoiding any foods that stimulate an inflammatory flare-up, add appropriate probiotics and gut lining support, and consider your adrenals—they are affected too. Nourish your body with bone marrow broth, gelatin, or protein shakes as tolerated and soups. Choose liquid-form foods that are nourishing and easy to digest.

Slowly add back each food group, one at a time and in small amounts. Try to rotate foods even though the list of food options can be severely limited for some. Should symptoms not improve with food eliminations and gut flora rebalancing, investigation of hidden infections and advanced food sensitivity testing is recommended.

A leaky gut and low-grade inflammation in the gut are big players in any gastrointestinal distress, thus herbal anti-inflammatories such as boswellia, turmeric, chewable licorice DGL, and goldenseal, along with other gut healing supplements are helpful to support your gut membrane integrity. I recommend using long-term leaky gut support with chronic Lyme; the infections, medications, and stress create a weakness in this area. Gelatin shakes with healthy fats can be helpful to maintain gut lining integrity. Refer to chapter seven for more information regarding gut healing and chapter twelve for a discussion on wide-ranging food challenges.

3. ELECTROLYTE REPLENISHMENT

Every function in the body is closely connected with major minerals, trace minerals, and electrolytes. With too-frequent or runny stools, the body looses excessive electrolytes and water. This creates organ stress, affecting the heart, brain, and kidneys, and exacerbates Lyme-related symptoms. Very low blood pressure, heart palpitations, excessive thirst, and hypoglycemia are also implicated with dehydration and a lack of electrolytes. In severe cases, chronic diarrhea with loss of electrolytes can lead to organ damage and shock. Alert your doctor when too-frequent elimination occurs.

Electrolyte replenishment is very helpful with too-frequent elimination. The primary minerals involved are potassium, magnesium, chloride, calcium, and sodium. They work in specific ratios with each other, and imbalances are linked to water retention in the body and blood pressure problems. A lack of electrolytes can manifest in various symptoms including muscle pain, worsened neurological symptoms, increased fatigue, and muscle cramping, all of which can mimic chronic Lyme symptoms. Not all symptoms are directly connected with chronic Lyme.

Vegetables and fruits such as cucumbers, leafy greens, beans, bananas, and avocados are loaded with potassium. Celery, beets, peppers, and sea salt contain sodium. Coconut water with potassium is helpful in a warm climate, but be sure to avoid the fruit juice sweetened ones. Sports drinks can contain great electrolyte mixes but many also contain added flavors and colors. With chronic stress, electrolytes are often already compromised, especially with severe dietary restrictions. When loose stools are an issue, add an electrolyte mix into your day (after discussing this with your doctor).

4. PALLIATIVE GREEN RELIEF

Green palliative relief options include using activated charcoal or bentonite clay throughout the day, until the excessive elimination calms down. These are binding agents that are effective and readily available without a prescription. Because they bind, be sure you do not take any charcoal or bentonite clay at the same time or too close to the time you take your medications or supplements. (At least two hours away).

Keep activated charcoal tablets, capsules, or powder in an airtight container—the powdered form will be more available because it does not have to be broken down. Both are also used for food poisonings and as binding agents during a detox cycle. In rare cases, charcoal can irritate the bowels. Discontinue use if that occurs.

Prescriptions from physicians often include cholestyramine, which is usually prescribed after gallbladder removal surgery to offset chronic diarrhea. It is best to get this from a compounded pharmacy, however, it is not recommended for long term use. Cholestyramine is also prescribed to support detox in mold-associated illnesses. Do follow your doctor's instructions if you are using cholestyramine.

Chlorella, cilantro, and spirulina are rich in chlorophyll and can be supportive in detox with binding agents, such as activated charcoal or bentonite clay. Food-based antioxidant powders can be helpful as liquefied supplementation, especially with challenged digestion. Powdered sources from whole foods can include rosehips, carrot root, green tea, acai, or pomegranate.

5. GUT FLORA REBALANCING AND HEALING A LEAKY GUT

Probiotics are very helpful for gut healing and essential with runny stools. Besides improving gut flora balance probiotics downshift histamine reactions and diarrhea-like symptoms. Imbalances and a lack of diversity in the gut flora are key contributing factors to overly frequent bowel movements. These can be induced by the infection or follow-up drug treatment, in addition to irritating foods and chronic psychological and emotional stress.

Probiotics, spores, or soil-based organisms must be introduced slowly; certain strains can actually make matters worse, causing severe bloating and constipation or possibly provoking a detox reaction (e.g., headaches, increased fatigue, gas, bloating, constipation, and nausea).

Certain clients respond well to probiotics in very high doses to repopulate the gut with certain strains after chronic antibiotic drug treatment. Do make a point to get out in nature and touch and feel the dirt. It is in the soil that health-supporting microbes propagate—an important factor in why it is good for children to play outside in a (organic) dirt-filled sandbox.

Healing the gut lining is very important; with the stress associated with chronic Lyme and related infections, gut lining integrity and the thickness of the membranes matter. It is part of our immune system. A healthier gut milieu will tone down its hyper-reactivity while its tolerance for all kinds of foods increases; this will lower inflammation in your body, and that will help you on your path toward wellness.

. . . .

Wrapping Up

It is easy to only think of ourselves only in the physical sense, yet we must remember that it is about the energy and vibrations in our body, including that of our trillions of microbes. If we are functioning with a low life force and engage in toxic thoughts and emotions at an energetic level, it will contribute to difficulties in recovering from Lyme-related infections.

"If you don't think your anxiety, depression, sadness, and stress impact your physical health, think again. All of these emotions trigger chemical reactions in your body, which can lead to inflammation and a weakened immune system. Learn how to cope, sweet friend. There will always be dark days."

—KRIS CARR

Chapter Eleven

The Mind-Body Connection

Take a quiet moment to look within; relax in a comfortable chair or yoga pose. It is with introspection that we can find clues and solutions to inner conflicts, while gaining clarity regarding troubling relationships or situations that keep us stuck psychologically and emotionally. What do we need to let go of? Could it be a belief, a toxic relationship, or inner anger at the infections that are keeping us sick? This is the deeper work that impacts our physiology, and it is something that you can do at home. Give your emotions space. Remember that you are more than a physical body.

The mind-body connection must be considered. The bowels and intestines are related to the first and second chakras, which are energetically connected to safety, security, financial matters, and relationships. Any concerns or insecurities in those areas will energetically manifest in the lower parts of the abdominal area, including the reproductive and the genital area. Were there emotional traumas, including loss of a parent or sexual abuse, during childhood? All these questions matter on an energetic level, because they will have physical manifestations.

If the mind is filled with anxiety, worry, and fear, the inner body feels like it is on a never-ending treadmill of stress without a stop or a pause button. The relentless worry and anxiety will manifest in a nervous digestive tract, indigestion, and too-frequent eliminations can be triggered. Mind-body calming techniques that address subconscious belief systems are helpful, but stress triggers must be investigated too. Professional coaching or therapy might be required, or consider healing modalities such as meditation, breathing exercises, and yoga that enable you to go within. Try to engage in creative activities that reduce your stress and give you joy.

Excessive worry will handicap the functions of the stomach, spleen, and pancreas, and with chronic *Borreliosis*, there is a lot to worry about. Fear, anger, and anxiety are all part of this scenario too; you have probably experienced years of not being understood, misdiagnosed, and perhaps were made to feel that you were not sick at all, or not "that" sick. You knew you were ill, even though the labs were negative or inconclusive. All these emotions constrict the natural flow of kidney, liver, and colon function.

Shame and guilt are toxic emotions. Repressing them will prevent you from becoming well. It is important to heal emotionally, to release hidden trauma, and to learn to love, live, and forgive. Many with persistent Lyme are angry and frustrated by physicians and others who do not understand their illness. Carrying anger in the heart and soul will not support a path to wellness; instead, it can often induce a spiral to depression and hopelessness. For many, it is helpful to read inspirational books that address deeper layers of emotional healing that offer a mind-set that is supportive during times of severe adversity. I recommend connecting with healing practitioners such as shamanic healers, energy workers, and medical intuitives.

We carry trauma, vulnerabilities, and wounds from the past four generations in our DNA. When we are exposed to unrelenting and terrifying stress, this state of fear will alter genes. These are passed on to the next four generations; consider genocide, fleeing a country, ongoing war, and colonization. Long-lasting effects of trauma and PTSD are being passed on along intergenerational lines through pregnancy. The research in this area, especially the work of neuroscientist Rachel Yehuda, has opened up an understanding of how prolonged stress affects a biochemical pathway called *methylation,* which is active in silencing harmful genes or turns them on. The structure of the gene is not altered, but its *function* is. This affects our ability to handle adversity in our lives and our overall constitution, including the strength and resilience of our immune system.

Disruptions in maternal care after pregnancy are also important in the predisposition and vulnerability of PTSD in childhood development and adult life when exposed to trauma, infections, environmental exposures, and mental stress. Low birth weight after the mother has been exposed to severe stress and trauma in the second and third trimester has been linked to behavioral and psychiatric problems. This was studied in pregnant women exposed to the attacks of September 11 in New York City.[1] Another well-known example includes maternal Holocaust survivors who have passed their PTSD to the next generation. Their children and grandchildren exhibit altered stress hormones.[2]

When living with Lyme, it is important to connect with living relatives to find out more about their lives, their traumas, their living environment with its challenges and fears, and their physical wounds. If possible, find out what happened in your parents lives while you were in the womb. Your mom's feelings and life challenges impact your ability to become well today. Your grandmother's grief and loss over the death of a child at childbirth might be keeping you from becoming well. This is an exciting new field in research. Hypnosis and Family Constellations are powerful tools to interrupt the intergenerational trauma and emotional wounds.

Often, a toxic mind-set or limiting subconscious belief systems are also in play, and they can contribute to your ongoing challenges. We are more than just a body with a head; our thoughts and emotions matter a great deal. Traumatic events in our present life, even traumas from past lives, play a role in our physiology as they become embedded in our DNA. Post-traumatic stress disorder (PTSD) is now much more prevalent, and it is not just occurring with soldiers returning from the wars abroad. Abuse of any kind, at any age, will be reflected in the body, weakening it even more.

It is at this psychological, emotional, and energetic level that homeopathy, essential oils, and flower essences shine. There is a great deal that we know, but there is also so much we do not know. These healing remedies eavesdrop on the disharmony, chaos, and emotional wounds (also known as *myasms*) that affect our mind-body wellness. At a vibrational and energetic level, they reestablish communication between organs and glands, restoring the body's innate ability to heal. Nature, too, allows us to energize with its colors, aromas, and sounds. Listening, smelling, breathing, and being present in the abundance of nature will lift the spirit and the body's resilience.

Another stress-reducing and healing application is Emotional Freedom Technique (EFT). It involves voicing positive and loving affirmations in conjunction with a gentle and repetitive tapping action on the meridians that are used in traditional acupuncture. Various tapping points include the top of the head, the area under the eyes, the side of the head, the collarbone, under the nose, in the hollow under the lips, under the arms, and the inside wrists. Firm tapping in these areas with the finger tips while integrating breath also stimulates the nerve endings in the fingers. You can do it yourself, in the comfort of your own home; it does not hurt, and it does not involve swallowing another pill. Make sure you are well hydrated before tapping. Electricity and energy in our body moves and communicates in the presence of water. There are multiple resources online, including practitioners that can provide professional guidance. These are a couple examples of a vocal affirmation:

"Even though I have . . . , I deeply and completely accept myself," or

"Even though I have this anger toward the Lyme, I deeply and completely accept myself."

It is important to only affirm what resonates and is comfortable for you. Simple tapping with the fingertips helps to clear energetic blockages by acknowledging the problem you are dealing with and instilling self-acceptance, instead of struggle and resistance, in the body—if you carefully tune in. Cognitive shifts can occur when reframing perceptions that are detrimental to your health, and these shifts can support you during the many tough times. It can become your "chill pill." At times, it might take more repetition for energies to shift.

What can you do to make changes for the better? See what resonates with you:

Mind-Body Connection Techniques to Support Your Healing Path

» Check off three of the following that you can realistically commit to.

☐ Meditate for ten minutes a day; choose a meditation app on your phone or a guided meditation on YouTube. As an alternative, practice ten minutes of EFT daily in your home.

☐ Sit under a tree, in nature, without looking at the phone. Instead, place conscious focus on the beauty of nature. Breathe and feel the healing power of nature.

☐ Commit to a weekly yoga class at home or at a studio near you. Start with twenty to thirty minutes; you do not want to be sore or excessively tired. Pace yourself.

☐ Call someone you need to make amends with who has been on your mind. Emotional burdens can weigh us down, and they lower our immune function.

☐ Join a mastermind group or other supportive business group to inspire your self-development.

☐ Read a page or one chapter a day in an inspirational book, such as *Daring Greatly* by Brene Brown, *Feelings Buried Alive Never Die* by Karol K. Truman, *Inviting A Monkey To Tea* by Nancy Collier, or *The Work* by Byron Katie.

☐ Consult with a Body Talk or Psych-K practitioner. Deep-seated belief systems and the subconscious mind must be addressed.

☐ Listen to classical music on your commute to work—maybe even hum along.

☐ Take time for introspection. This is a time without judgment, a time for being accountable, and a time of making peace with an inner ongoing struggle—a time for gratitude.

· · · · · · ·

Wrapping Up

We must address wellness one day at a time. You might have disagreed with me here and there, and that is OK. My goal is to present you with an array of holistic options that include structured action steps to guide you along the way; it is your choice to implement strategies that resonate with you and are appropriate for you. I am fully aware that with these persistent infections, there are many degrees of sickness symptoms, with good days and bad days. We are all on our own path in this life. I am also aware that when you are sick, there is only so much you can do or implement, even if you wish you could do more. Just by reading this book, or a few pages, you are doing something to help your future health. I just hope that you are not going it alone. If you do not have support at home, seek out a healing community.

Client education is a big part of my work, and a personalized approach is key to improving my client's wellness while they are in active or nonactive Lyme treatment. I interact with Lyme-literate Medical Doctors and am fully aware of the long waiting times. You are welcome to arrange a consultation to discuss your specific nutritional and health-supporting needs with me.

Commercial health and cookie-cutter nutritional coaching is not appropriate in chronic Lyme and coinfection cases. With late-diagnosed Lyme, secondary underlying infections, chronic inflammation, digestive troubles, and often multiple drug interventions, the terrain is severely compromised. Multiple biological systems must slowly be supported concurrently with customized nutrition, a lifestyle assessment, stress reduction techniques, digestive restoration, reduction of toxic environmental exposures, and opening of elimination pathways.

Any acute crisis must be dealt with, and it might require taking a few steps back. Slow and steady progress is important, but it will not be linear. It is most important to listen to your body; it knows best, and it will be responsive when you give it the chance to do so.

Teamwork is imperative to ensure the best long-term outcome for the chronic Lyme patient. It is my desire to complement and collaborate with Lyme-literate physicians to facilitate improved resilience, function, and quality of life for the individual who has been on a long, misunderstood, and often lonely road of illness.

For many, a multi-faceted and integrated approach facilitates improved energy and resilience, happier moods, and energy to engage on a social level. This approach gives hope that a better life is possible for many when living with persistent Lyme. You were born with unlimited potential.

> "You were born with goodness and trust.
> You were born with ideals and dreams.
> You were born with greatness.
> You were born with wings.
> You are not meant for crawling, so don't.
> You have wings.
> Learn to use them and fly."
>
> —RUMI

Chapter Twelve

"Friend or Foe" Foods

You are unique in your dietary needs. In this chapter, we will go into detail about food groups that might be giving you health troubles—even though they are known as healthy foods.

Traditional food preparation, including soaking, fermentation, stone grinding, preserving, and slow cooking, have very much given way to instant or frozen meals, commercially processed foods, pasteurization, deep frying, and microwaving.

Salt, sugar, gluten, and unhealthy fats are mainstays of the Standard American Diet. This has contributed to alterations in our intestinal ecosystem, diversity of microbes, and our taste buds. We know now that certain microbes in the gut contribute to sugar and fat cravings. The 100 trillion microbes play an important role in controlling eating behavior, leptin and insulin levels, satiety, and obesity; they also manipulate moods.[1] Overgrowth of any species of microbe occurs at the expense of our wellness and mental health. This was discovered over a hundred years ago, yet it is not considered in conventional psychiatry or internal medicine.

With digestive troubles, examine your current diet and take note of any food groups you eat of lot of on a regular, even daily, basis. For example, in the summer, are you consuming a lot of peppers, tomatoes, and eggplant that might be a pain trigger for you? Or do you add banana and avocado into your daily shake, and it makes you feel bloated? Maybe you have been eating a lot of garlic, because it supports the immune system, but you have been experiencing severe gas and constipation.

Are you overindulging in almond butter because it is healthy? Or are you eating too much fruit that can increase your joint pain? Maybe you are on a severely restricted diet right now; could you do a little better with food preparation to help the digestive system? Perhaps you did not realize that the balsamic vinaigrette you like is causing your headaches or bloating.

Even if food modifications are essential in the beginning when living with Lyme and all its complexities, the long-term goal is to develop an immune system that will become tolerant of many different foods. Preparing fresh foods at home and cooking meals that are shared with loved ones will support nourishment and healing on many levels—well beyond the food.

Diverse foods = diverse microbiome = improved energy, mood, and health = resilience.

Everyone is different, and in today's world there are many trendy dietary viewpoints that can be very confusing. It is difficult to prove nutrition through science. How you react to kale or goat kefir will be different than the way I or your best friend react to it.

To give you a broader landscape of possible food triggers that are possible obstacles in your path to wellness, consider the following information.

The High-Histamine Food Factor

If when you get bitten by mosquitoes or other bugs you have severe skin or itching reactions or you get frequent headaches or you have estrogen dominance with PMS and fibroids, you might want to consider this important factor: We all have different levels of histamine, and they fluctuate throughout the day; thus, it is not easy to test histamine levels in the blood.

Histamine is a brain chemical, or neurotransmitter, that is a messaging molecule. It occurs naturally in plants and animals. We need it to help our bodies function in many ways. Histamine was discovered in 1911 as a major player in allergic diseases, and it is involved in vital actions such as the production of stomach acid and the lowering of blood pressure. It is also a chemical messenger in the brain, and it causes a runny nose when we have a cold or allergies as the immune system is trying to get rid of perceived environmental threats. Histamine is also a pro-inflammatory constrictor of smooth muscle; it tightens muscles in the brain, heart, gut, throat, and lungs. This matters in illnesses such as asthma, anaphylaxis with nuts or bee stings, Crohn's disease, and irritable bowel syndrome.

What many do not know is that the gut produces the greatest amount of histamine. If there is a histamine problem, there is a gut issue. Prescription medications such as H2 blockers, proton pump inhibitors (acid blockers), anti-depressants, opioids, and antibiotics adversely affect the gut flora, the mucosal lining of the gut, and specific enzymes involved in histamine degradation.[2] It accumulates in the blood stream.

We need histamine, but we do not want too much of it in our bloodstream. Individuals with intestinal permeability, translocation of microbes in the intestines, lack of stomach acid, and certain genetic predispositions can have difficulty breaking down histamine; this is connected with a specific enzyme, diamine oxidase. It might have been an underlying health concern since childhood already, and medical history can provide clues in this regard. Elevated levels of histamine in the bloodstream causes reactions to foods that contain high levels of histamine, alcohol, chemical exposures, mold, and other environmental triggers.

But it is not just about food, the gut, and environmental allergens; it is also about estrogen. Female hormones play an important role in allergic diseases such as asthma, especially in regards to mast cell activity. Menstrual cycles and elevated estrogen levels have been shown to be interlinked with histamine-related challenges; thus, it is even more complex for girls and women. When living with Lyme, we must address the whole person. It is not just about the infections anymore: Various biological and hormonal functions are severely compromised.[3] During pregnancy, though, levels of the DAO enzymes increase and histamine-related symptoms decrease until the child is born.

Too much accumulated histamine creates havoc in the body, contributing to IBS, mast cell disorders, chronic diarrhea, migraines, and glutamate disorders. If you are very allergic, have itchy skin, or your skin swells up abnormally with a mosquito bite, elevated histamine may be an issue for you. Whole blood histamine (not serum histamine) is the blood marker that can be tested, but it must be seen in context with clinical symptoms as blood levels fluctuate during the day.

Certain foods contain higher levels of histamine, and these can make any allergy, salicylate, or histamine-related symptom worse, including PMS, runny nose, headaches, diarrhea, low blood pressure, hives, asthma, rheumatoid arthritis, psychotic episodes, and even anaphylaxis. Do know it is the bacteria in the foods that produce histamine as their natural metabolic by-product. Common foods that are high in histamine include the following:

- Aged, pickled, or fermented foods such as kombucha, alcohol, vinegar, or cheese
- Cured or smoked meats
- Canned food
- Seafood
- Avocado
- Eggplant
- Spinach
- Tomato
- Dried fruits
- Mushrooms

In addition, there are foods that encourage the release of histamine from mast cells, which are like storage tanks for histamine in various areas of the body, including the skin, mouth, lungs, nose, and intestines. Foods that can prompt release of histamine from mast cells include citrus fruits, papaya, pineapples, nuts, strawberries, egg whites, and additives.

The mast cells release histamine when you eat certain foods but also when exposed to certain substances, chemicals, or pets. This provokes an allergic reaction such as itching, sneezing, or headaches, and even psychiatric symptoms, which are often misdiagnosed. It can also provoke the itchiness you feel when a wound on the skin is healing as part of the natural healing process.

Genetic testing is a helpful way to check for predispositions regarding histamine and the ability to metabolize it efficiently; however, genes cannot be treated, and they are not diagnostic. Instead, genetic predispositions in conjunction with clinical findings (and symptoms) can be modulated with targeted nutrients. Skin prick testing through a doctor is an option, but it is not very accurate for many. 23andMe is a genetic saliva test that checks for genetic variants and potential histamine risk factors.

Eating fresh foods is important because aged foods contain more histamine. As enzymes degrade cooked foods, especially leftover animal proteins, they increase in histamine. When cooking, store or freeze leftovers quickly to prevent increasing histamine in the aging process. Fresh fish and meats, vegetables, quinoa, rice, leafy herbs, coconut products, and healthy oils are all lower in histamine.

When symptoms that can be indicative of possible histamine excess are present, challenges with the small bowel enterocytes and gut flora imbalances must be addressed.[4] These modulate the body's immune and inflammatory response when exposed to high histamine foods, such as vinegars or alcohol that might have been added unknowingly to foods. Additives, artificial colors, and preservatives in foods can trigger acute histamine-related symptoms, including headaches, breathing difficulties, and hyperexcitable behavior.

In addition, support from DAO enzymes that break down histamine, anti-inflammatories, immune modulating and liver cleansing supplementation is helpful. You might consider keeping DAO inhibitor enzymes in your bag to protect against accidental high-histamine exposures when eating out. One of my favorite supplement choices with histamine-related challenges is Antronex from Standard Process. There are various DAO blocking supplements available today.

The spice turmeric and the anti-inflammatory plant flavonoid, or quercetin, can be helpful at higher doses against mast cell activation; thus, it is also helpful with seasonal allergies. Quercetin is found in capers, onions, asparagus, dark red or blue fruits and vegetables, such as blueberries, and some lettuces. Cooking does not destroy histamine.

The Dairy Factor

It is best to eliminate dairy, especially with gluten sensitivity, migraines, respiratory challenges, SIBO, autism and other spectrum–related issues, neurological symptoms, chronic vaginal yeast infections, thrush in the mouth or skin, or colon and upper respiratory health challenges.

Dairy products, especially pasteurized cow milk products, are inflammatory and produce mucus. They also have a morphine-like effect on the brain, which

I mentioned earlier in the book. Increased mucus production is undesirable for many because it paves the way for opportunistic bacterial infections to occur.

If you tolerate sheep or goat dairy products (e.g., cheese, yogurt, kefir, cottage cheese, and butter) rotate various dairy products to offset sensitivities. Individuals from European descent seem to tolerate milk better—ancestry does matter when it comes to food tolerance. With cultured milk products, the naturally occurring yeast, or lactase, feeds on the sugar in milk. This gets neutralized during the fermentation process, resulting in sour milk or kefir with immune-modulating microbes, especially *Lactobacillus*.[5] Raw dairy has terrific health benefits if tolerated; however, it is not an option for many, and it must come from a clean source.

Today, there are many milk substitutes. Coconut milk, rice milk, or one of the nut milks may be good alternatives in some cases, even though they are processed foods that contain additives. They often contain carrageenan, a known gut irritant, which is extracted from red seaweed. Be sure you read the labels. I call these caution foods. If you choose to use these milk substitutes, choose the ones without added sugars or flavors. If almonds or Brazil nuts are tolerated, you might consider making your own nut milk at home that is free from preservatives and processing. There are great sites online that give step-by-step video instructions.

Avoid low-fat, ultra-pasteurized milk, skim milk, soy milk, nondairy creamers, and imitation dairy or cheese products—even if organic. Many are by-products from processing and are considered dead foods. If they are fortified, they are dead foods to begin with.

The Oxalates Factor

Oxalates occur naturally as an inner defense in plants, yet they are highly reactive and inflammatory molecules that also result from metabolic processes in our body. Oxalates are naturally found in the environment, and they are also released offensively by harmful infections in the body (e.g., mold and *Candida*).

Foods that are high in oxalates include soy, beet greens, rhubarb, parsley, spinach, Swiss chard, and cocoa. Individuals who follow a plant-based diet with daily consumption of spinach, soy, and nuts, or use high-oxalate vegetables for daily juicing, greatly increase their susceptibility to kidney stones. Foods that are lower in oxalates include broccoli, berries, leeks, green beans, celery, apples, lettuce, carrots, kale, and parsnips.

A healthy body can break down and remove excess oxalates. However, with chronic Lyme-related and toxic mold infections, intestinal barrier dysfunction (leaky gut), and malnourishment, oxalates accumulate in the body—and then they are difficult to eliminate. Oxalates from foods are associated with increased inflammation and various health symptoms, including chronic yeast infections, kidney stones, osteoporosis, Spectrum-related symptoms, neurological and behavioral challenges, vulvodynia, and fibromyalgia.

Insufficient hydrochloric acid in the stomach will adversely affect the absorption of calcium, zinc, and magnesium from foods. These, in conjunction with arginine, vitamin B6 (in the form of P5P), and molybdenum, assist in breaking down excessive oxalate accumulation in the body. Elevated levels of free copper and iron make matters worse.

A gut flora that is out of balance compounds oxalate-related symptoms. Antibiotics kill off a certain beneficial gut microbe, *O. formigenes*, which is supposed to neutralize the excess oxalates. Low levels, or if it is nonexistent, of this gut microbe, plus elevated oxalates and *Candida* infections, are found in many children diagnosed on the Autism spectrum.

The oxalates, in the form of sharp crystals, can create internal irritation of membranes and increase inflammation, leading to joint pain. The buildup of calcium oxalates can contribute to oxalate arthritis, a painful condition affecting the joints that can be a factor in tendon damage. Calcium and oxalate crystals are also implicated in the painful inflammatory condition called *pseudogout*; actual gout is indicated by the buildup of uric acid crystals in the joints. *Aspergillus*, or black mold, in the home contributes to oxalate crystal buildup found in chronic sinusitis, interstitial cystitis, and lung infections.

Oxalates deplete glutathione, adversely affecting the body's ability to detox heavy metals and other toxins. In the body, oxalates bind to lead and mercury, preventing excretion of these toxic metals. The individual will be more symptomatic. The Organic Acids Test from Great Plains is helpful in discerning oxalate challenges.

If you are eating a diet high in oxalates and are already implementing severe food eliminations, you might consider decreasing foods that are high in oxalates, tapering their consumption down slowly over a few months. You do not want to stop abruptly because this can bring on a severe detox reaction.

If the above resonates with you and you are experiencing symptoms that might be connected to oxalates, focus on eliminating simple sugars and foods that contain yeast first to reduce the internal fungal overgrowth. Integrate herbal teas and foods that are not on the high-oxalate list, and make sure you are supplementing with a good vitamin B complex, calcium citrate, magnesium, and bile salts or Swedish bitters. Omega-3 fatty acids, cod liver oil, calcium citrate, and magnesium are helpful to reduce oxalate absorption in the intestines. When living with Lyme, consider a lower oxalate diet and see if you feel change for the better.

Keep working on the gut by making sure your probiotic contains *B. lactis* and *Lactobacillus acidophilus,* both of which assist in degrading oxalates in the intestine. We must always look at the big picture of nutritional deficiencies, underlying infections, heavy metal toxicities, and the overall health of the gut.[6]

The Salicylates Factor

Salicylates are potent natural plant toxins and preservatives, which plants use for protection against diseases and predators. These plant toxins have a medicinal effect, just like over-the-counter pain-relieving and anti-inflammatory drugs that are synthesized forms of a compound isolated from the bark of the white willow tree. Salicylate sensitivity or intolerance can occur with synthetic and natural forms of salicylates including medications, perfumes, preservatives, and foods. Symptoms can include respiratory allergy symptoms, asthma, hives, irritable bowel syndrome, colitis, mucus production, and dilated blood vessels contributing to low blood pressure. Many symptoms associated with salicylate intolerance can also mimic Lyme-related symptoms.

If you have already embarked on multiple food eliminations and antimicrobial gut programs, yet are still experiencing digestive or allergy-like ailments, consider decreasing salicylate exposure from foods. It is the cumulative effect of these that can tip the scale in a compromised gut. A three-week restriction of foods high in salicylates can be done as a self-test, to see if there is symptom relief of any kind. Currently, there is no lab test or skin test available, yet an unknown salicylate sensitivity is an additional challenge for many. You will notice in the examples below that some high-salicylate vegetables are part of the nightshade family, so it can be a double whammy of plant toxins if the gut is compromised.

Peel vegetables well before cooking; only eat ripe vegetables and fruits when their salicylate content is lower. Check out the foods in the table that follows; you might be surprised that these foods are deemed healthy.

High-Salicylate Vegetables	Moderate-Salicylate Vegetables	High-Salicylate Oils	Fruits Low in Salicylates
Cooked tomatoes	Asparagus	Coconut	Golden Delicious Apples
Broccoli	Beets	Olive	Limes
Cucumber	Potatoes	Sesame	Pears
Zucchini	Mushrooms	Walnut	Papaya
Spinach	Carrots		Bananas
Sweet potatoes			
Eggplant			
Chili peppers			
Alfalfa sprouts			

SOURCE: HTTP://WWW.WESTONAPRICE.ORG/HEALTH-TOPICS/PLANTS-BITE-BACK/

Remember, multiple food sensitivities and digestive troubles will subside when you take care of infections in the gut, increase the diversity of the flora, and heal the gut lining—but it takes time. It may even take years, especially with Lyme-related infections if medications are still in play. It is not about the food; it is about how your gut responds to the food.

Grains, Root Vegetables, and Sugars

FRIEND?

When eating healthy higher-glycemic and starchy foods, such as rice, amaranth, yams, squashes, creamed buckwheat, or quinoa, make sure to add a protein source and a healthy fat to the meal. When eaten alone, these foods perpetuate blood sugar swings associated with persistent Lyme. With their higher sugar content, they might not be appropriate for individuals dealing with fungal infections initially, yet that must be assessed on an individual basis.

Traditional cultures prepared grains for consumption by methods that included soaking, sprouting, grinding, and air fermentation. It took hard work and a few days to create a loaf of bread from flour, water, and air. The various processes neutralized inhibiting plant enzymes, or phytic acid, while retaining the full array of fiber and nutrients, including the wheat germ or rice germ. The body is able to digest these carefully prepared and simple ingredients. With traditional food preparation, B vitamins including niacin and folate and minerals such as magnesium, zinc, and iron are all made bioavailable. These nutrients are lacking in processed grains today. Instead, many ingredients and synthesized vitamins and folic acid are added as fortification, but the body knows the difference. It has a difficult time digesting processed foods that induce inflammation.

Root vegetables have an array of health benefits. They contain phytonutrients that nourish our spleen and kidneys as well as encourage blood building, especially when we are not well. We need robust blood to facilitate oxygen transport and give us energy. We need immune support when the body is challenged by chronic infections, and these foods provide energetic and nutrient fortification for the body.

Orange and red root vegetables are nutrient dense in beta-carotene, which supports our eyes, skin, and immune system. When cooked, these vegetables are known as warming foods that aid our bodies during cold winter months and help our digestion. They are health supporting when tough digestive challenges requiring a specific, low complex-carbohydrate diet, but they must be buffered with protein and fat to stabilize blood sugar. Blood sugar imbalances are always of great concern with chronic Lyme, vagus nerve disruption, and POTS (dysautonomia).

It is important to distinguish between processed or refined sugars and naturally occurring sugars. There is a big difference, and, again, we must not forget the wisdom of traditional cultures in which some whole food sources of naturally occuring sugars, such as raw honey or molasses or a piece of fruit, were prized for their sweetness. In Chinese medicine, sweetness is important because it enhances digestion, health, and well-being, especially with prolonged stress.

When living with Lyme, consumption of sugars can quickly spike your blood sugar, especially if it is refined sugar, which does not contain fiber. At the start of a meal, eat some protein before consuming higher sugar vegetables or whole grains. Fiber slows the blood sugar spike; however, these are caution foods for some. With Lyme and hypoglycemia, it is essential to buffer these foods with healthy fats and proteins at every meal.

There are various trendy diets out there, and some severely limit the intake of carbohydrates and sugars of all kinds. How we metabolize carbohydrates, fruits, and sugars is different for each of us. This can be assessed with the Healthexcel system of Metabolic Typing. Many ill individuals do not tolerate an exclusionary diet of high protein and high fat in the long term, and they end up with hypoglycemia, adrenal dysregulation, thyroid trouble, and energy crashes. On the flip side, the consumption of sugar-laden processed foods leads to an increase in type 2 diabetes and obesity, and that is alarming. Refined sugar is addictive and can cause severe sugar and carb cravings.

We all enjoy and need some sweetness in our lives, especially when dealing with prolonged health problems, including challenges with chronic fatigue (mitochondrial dysfunction), cognition, sleep, pain, and digestion; thus, a sweet treat has its place. Options for naturally occurring sugars include a little raw honey in oatmeal, stewed or baked fruit, a cookie made with coconut sugar, hot chocolate made with almond or coconut milk, or apple sauce with stevia. There are natural options, and it is best to avoid refined sugars that spike blood sugars and contribute to hypoglycemia, insulin resistance, and weight gain.

Sugars feed infections and harmful microbes; use your own judgment on what is best for you. Stevia can be used as a sweetener; however, not everyone tolerates it well. Root vegetables and fruits can provide needed sweetness. Let us also consider that a little sweetness at the end of the meal actually helps digestion. If tolerated, a stewed apple, warm applesauce with stevia and cinnamon, licorice root tea, a little kefir with local raw honey, or a piece of dark organic chocolate are some healthy options to meet the need for something sweet.

FOE?

Grains have inflammatory properties that can lead to intestinal permeability (leaky gut) and a leaky brain, which increases neurological pain and nerve-related symptoms. It is best to avoid all grains with severe Lyme-related neurological health challenges, brain fog, and chronic joint pain. Also, grains (in particular gluten, rice, and millet) can contribute to chronic constipation or too-frequent eliminations that are associated with secondary gut infections including SIBO, irritable bowel syndrome, diverticulitis, ulcerative colitis, and Crohn's disease. If the gut is not well and certain genetics are in play, grains are best avoided. Listen to your body.

Plant toxins in grains, legumes, nuts, and seeds are called *phytates*. These protect the plant against early germination and store the phosphorous the plant requires to grow. To deactivate phytic acid, the grains, legumes, and nuts are best prepared in a warm, moist, and slightly acidic medium. Soak grains (and legumes) overnight in a bowl filled with water and sea salt or raw apple cider vinegar to neutralize the phytic acid. Rinse well in the morning and dry naturally. With legumes, this might require repeated cycles over twenty-four hours.

Phytate enzyme inhibitors block the absorption of nutrients such as zinc, iron, B vitamins, and calcium, which are essential for immune system health. A lack of iron is associated with fatigue; beans are not very good sources of iron to begin with, and absorption of what iron they do contain is low. Zinc is required for over three hundred enzyme activities, yet cannot be absorbed from foods if they are not properly prepared. All of these considerations matter when dealing with chronic Lyme infections.

Plant toxins also include lectins. These are also found in grains, beans, and soybeans. A healthy gut can neutralize this plant toxin, but a compromised, leaky gut will not be able to break down the lectins efficiently, and they can contribute to damage and inflammation in the small intestine in addition to affecting brain function. Digestive enzymes are helpful.

Once in the bloodstream, lectins can induce allergies, sensitivities, mood disorders, altered gut flora, and increased blood viscosity. With Lyme infections and genetic variations (including C677T), increased blood viscosity can already be of concern.

Nightshade Vegetables

FRIEND?

Oh, the joys of summer! Tomatoes, potatoes, peppers (including cayenne and paprika), and eggplant are well-known nightshade plants. With their red, orange, yellow, and purple colors, they provide great sources of phytonutrients. They are abundant in naturally occurring antioxidants, vitamins, minerals, carotenoids, and fiber. Other nightshades include goji berries, pepinos, pimentos, ashwagandha, and naranjillas; all these have health benefits, too. Each color and vegetable corresponds to an organ in the body. Thus, at an energetic level, these multicolored vegetables and fruits nourish the organs, including the spleen, liver, heart, and digestive system, but they are not for everyone.

Nightshades are great sources of potassium, vitamin C, and lycopene, especially tomatoes and multiple varieties of peppers. Cayenne is known to assist capillary dilation and circulation in colder climates, yet many cannot tolerate it and can experience a severe reaction with accidental exposure. Pureed tomato sauce in a jar is a great source of lycopene.

If you tolerate nightshade fruits and vegetables, buy them freshly picked from an organic or local farmer to avoid the GMOs and pesticide overload associated with commercial produce. An alternative is to buy organic frozen vegetables and fruits. It is best to consume these vegetables ripe and when they are in season because they are highest in desirable nutrients then, with lower plant toxins. It is best not to eat them every day; add them into a food rotation to offset any low-grade inflammation associated with nightshades.

FOE?

Nightshades use toxins called *trypsins* like an internal bug spray to protect themselves against predators, including insects and herbivores (and us!). Nightshade vegetables also contain innate plant toxins; alkaloids are one type of plant toxin. Species of the nightshade family include cayenne pepper, chili pepper, ground red pepper, crushed red pepper, curry, and paprika. When cooking, prepare these nightshade vegetables well to neutralize the trypsin inhibitors that prevent absorption of plant nutrients.

Trypsin and alkaloids can add an inflammatory burden for some individuals. They can severely increase joint pain with autoimmune and Lyme-related joint diseases. Gut health, of course, comes into play because a compromised gut may have decreased tolerance for the plant toxins, yet joint pain must also be seen in context with the Lyme infection. Thus, the cumulative buildup of infectious and plant toxins creates additional immune system irritation and concomitant inflammation that leaves joints swollen and painful.

Rotating foods is helpful to prevent an overload of foods in your system that might, unbeknownst to you, irritate your body and worsen your Lyme-related symptoms. You might be able to handle a few tomatoes once a week or a potato here and there, but maybe not all together or that often. It is never just one food that causes trouble. There are always multiple factors in play, and that can make it difficult to discern where to make changes. You can do a self-test elimination of all nightshades for three weeks to determine if there is any change for the better in your joint pain and other symptoms. If you omit nightshades and you have less arthritic pains in your joints, there is your answer. You could try to reintroduce them occasionally, one at a time; however, if your symptoms flare, it might be best to avoid them all together.

Yeasts

FRIEND?

Yeasts and fungi are part of a healthy soil ecosystem, if they are kept in check—it is the same in the gut. Yeast is a one-celled fungus; they are an important part of nature's ecosystem. In nature, yeasts live in symbiotic relationship with plants.

They provide immune protection against threats. Their toxins are a plant's own antibiotic against harmful microbes in the soil. (Fungal toxins are used in chemotherapy and for immune suppression in patients with organ transplants.)

There are over two hundred known yeasts, and many of them are beneficial; they are a great source of amino acids, minerals, and vitamins. Beta glucans from the walls of brewer's yeast and nutritional yeast extract are well known for their immune-boosting properties.

Activated or dry yeasts have been used as fermentation agents in baking, alcohol production, and biofuel production. Nutritional yeast, a deactivated yeast, is grown on beet sugar. It is a great source of folate and other B vitamins, especially vitamin B12. It assists with production of red blood cells and is high in protein. It is vegetarian-based.

Supplementation with health-supporting and gut-friendly yeasts is very helpful for many during antibiotic treatment. The goal is to use these yeast strains to crowd out harmful opportunistic yeast or fungus that is often present with a weakened immune system or mercury toxicity. Yeasts such as *Saccharomyces cerevisiae* and *Saccharomyces boulardii* are used in therapeutic programs to help restore microbial balance in the gut, especially with prolonged antibiotic use or after surgery. *S. boulardii* is also very helpful when dealing with a debilitating *C. difficile* infection.

FOE?

With yeast infections (acute or chronic), it is best to avoid sugars, dairy, and yeast-containing foods that feed the out-of-control fermentation process in the gut. This includes high-sugar foods, bread, alcohol, fermented vinegars, baker's and brewer's yeast, starches, root vegetables, and high-sugar fruits—even nutritional supplements that contain yeasts. Fermented vegetables work well for some, yet others experience a worsening of symptoms when consuming fermented foods. High histamine and high oxalates are blocking factors that should also be considered.

Chronic Lyme and its immune-suppressing properties often open the door for chronic fungal infections. Pharmaceutical agents such as nystatin or fluconazole are often used; however, yeast overgrowth soon returns, especially with long-term use of antibiotic medications, adrenal fatigue, thyroid challenges, heavy metal toxicity, sleep troubles, and chronic life stress. Exposures to mold in the environment will worsen symptoms and inflammation with a hyperactive immune response.

An overgrowth of harmful yeasts creates a great challenge for the immune system; its toxins are powerful, and they contribute to brain fog, joint pain, and systemic inflammation.

Fruits

FRIEND?

Fruits are a great source of bioflavonoids, carotenoids, lycopene, and other antioxidants, and they provide an array of vitamins, minerals, and fiber. Generally, berries, cranberries, and cherries are great for the kidneys; bananas provide potassium and inulin (prebiotic fiber); and avocados are a source of healthy and delicious fat. The skin and flesh of fruits offer a good source of fiber, water, and electrolytes (e.g., the potassium in a watermelon). Their fiber lowers the blood sugar impact from the natural fruit sugar, or fructose. It is always best to eat, not drink, fruit. Sugars are concentrated in juice and the fiber is low or entirely absent. I recommend eating only fruit that is in season, buying local, and going organic. And do grate lemon or orange peel over salads.

FOE?

Raw fruits are cooling foods. They can contribute to indigestion by fermenting in the stomach. Fruits contain fructose, which can cause increased joint inflammation, feed infections, elevated uric acid levels, and is a major contributor to gout. (You can read about fruits in the section on oxalates and salicylates.)

The peel of fruits can be very difficult to digest, especially if the digestive tract is compromised from drug treatments and hidden gastrointestinal infections. The fiber in fruits can aggravate underlying gut issues, especially in connection with SIBO. Avoid commercial fruits; they are sprayed up to forty-five times with pesticides, especially commercial strawberries. With compromised digestion and Lyme-associated blood sugar imbalances, it is best to eat only lower-glycemic organic fruits, and I recommend enjoying them either stewed or baked.

Citrus fruits are inflammatory for many and are best avoided with Lyme-related chronic arthritis pain and urinary tract symptoms.

Popular crushed iced fruit drinks in the hot summer months are best eliminated. They spike blood sugar and cause a constriction in an already challenged body. Cold or room-temperature drinks are best in hot summer months. You can create a spritzer infusion with sparkling water and a touch of lime, lemon, orange, mint, or watermelon (and stevia).

Dark Leafy Greens

FRIEND?

Dark green, leafy vegetables, or complex carbohydrates, include kale, collard greens, chard, and dandelion greens. They are nutrient-rich, low in sugars, and dense in fiber, especially when grown in healthy soil. As such, they are optimal carb choices for blood sugar balance, and they stimulate essential blood cleansing and blood building, which are so needed with chronic Lyme and mold-related illness.

Dark leafy greens are good sources of vitamins A, C, and K. They also contain a large amount of iron, which supports blood building and energy. With anemia, dark greens, including spirulina and chlorella, are helpful. (Liver provides the best source of iron but is not an option for some individuals). A tea with nettles or dandelion enhances drainage, kidney, and liver function, all of which are compromised with chronic Lyme and use of medications.

The bitterness in dark leafy greens helps stimulate digestion and gallbladder function. As a health practitioner, I always prefer to use a food-first approach. I recommend eating cooked dark leafy greens as a source of iron while also integrating them for blood cleansing and detoxification. I also like to add them into my smoothies to increase fiber and nutrient value, never raw. Some leafy greens are fairly bitter, such as winter kale, while others have a sweeter flavor, like rainbow chard. The addition of sautéed onions can sweeten the taste when cooking bitter leafy greens.

Dark leafy greens also provide bioavailable sources of folate and water-soluble vitamin B9, which is required for detoxification pathways and DNA protection in the body. Those pathways can be challenged with Lyme-related infection, and additional supplementation of methylfolate is helpful. Vegetables that are high in bioavailable folate include leafy greens such as Swiss chard, dandelion, mustard greens, watercress, escarole, spinach, asparagus, mustard greens, parsley, romaine lettuce, collard greens, lentils, and turnips.

FOE?

When secondary gastrointestinal infections such as SIBO are present, the high-fiber, dark leafy greens can make symptoms of gas, bloating, stomach pain, and constipation or diarrhea worse. Harmful bacteria in the gut can ferment the undigested fiber of these veggies, creating great digestive discomfort.

These vegetables are also rich in oxalates that can cause problems for certain individuals. Oxalate buildup is implicated in kidney stones, gout, vulvodynia, interstitial cystitis, and joint pains in the extremities. This is one good reason not to eat raw spinach or kale.

Boil, steam, or sauté all dark leafy greens to make the nutrients bioavailable and to neutralize oxalic acid that binds to the minerals and inhibits their absorption.

Cruciferous Vegetables

FRIEND?

Cruciferous vegetables, such as cabbages, cauliflower, broccoli, and brussels sprouts, are high in fiber and support the gut flora. Whole foods have an innate intelligence that supersedes any supplement; thus, you want to integrate these vegetables into your nutritional strategy. Cruciferous vegetables play an important role in supporting our detox pathways in the liver. These vegetables also provide anti-cancer protection by assisting the body to get rid of excess estrogens that are harmful for women, men, and children. In addition, they provide a great source of fiber.

Fermented cabbages such as sauerkraut are high in nutritional value as enzymes have made the food more bioavailable. Cabbage juice is helpful for stomach concerns and possibly loose bowels. Steam broccoli or cabbage and keep them in the fridge so they are ready to add to your soups or shakes in small amounts. Steam a head of cauliflower and mash it with some butter or coconut oil and sea salt for a low-glycemic, mashed cauliflower side dish to substitute for potatoes.

With any reproductive challenges, estrogen dominance, prostate concerns, and PMS-related symptoms, neutralizing chemical estrogens is vital. Sulfu-raphane is found in these vegetables, and it can metabolize the excess chemical estrogens, called *xenoestrogens*. Xenoestrogens are chemical estrogens in plastics, personal care products, and pesticides, and they contribute to cellular fatigue, abnormal cell growth, and hormonal disorders, making Lyme symptoms worse. The detox agent in cruciferous vegetables, called *sulforaphane*, helps the body to get rid of excess hormones in the liver. If you are able to digest these foods, add a variety into your daily meals—but not in raw form.

Sulforaphane content in cruciferous vegetables is reduced by cooking, and in many cases, supplementation is helpful. (It is actually created when you bite into the broccoli; an enzyme mixes with glucosinolate to create sulforaphane, kind of like the chemical reaction you get when you snap a glow stick.)

FOE?

These foods are known thyroid inhibitors, and Lyme infections may already play havoc with the thyroid gland. The plant toxins from cruciferous vegetables are called *goitrogens,* and they prevent the thyroid from absorbing iodine, a very important immune, reproductive health, and thyroid-supporting mineral. This also applies to dark leafy vegetables such as broccoli, bok choy, cabbages, kohl-rabi, and kale.

If large amounts of cruciferous vegetables are eaten or you already have low iodine levels, the thyroid will be more challenged in its daily functions, which includes temperature regulation, microcirculation in the hands and feet, the metabolic rate, mood, and more. An iodine deficiency challenge can contribute to swelling of the thyroid, called a *goiter,* and a hypothyroid condition. Sea salt does not offer sufficient levels of iodine, which is a popular belief. The iodine levels in iodized salt are sufficient to prevent a goiter, but they are not optimal to support the whole body's needs.

These foods are also high in easily-fermentable complex carbohydrates—the fermentable oligosaccharides, disaccharides, monosaccharides, and polyols (FOD-MAPS). Cruciferous vegetables must be severely restricted initially and properly prepared when various gut infections, including SIBO or IBS, are in play.

Because these vegetables are hard to digest, it is best not to eat them raw. They can create severe digestive discomfort, including bloating and smelly gas. Boil, sauté, or steam these vegetables before you eat them to neutralize plant toxins that affect thyroid function adversely. If you do add kale to your smoothie, steam or blanch it first to improve absorption and to neutralize toxins.

Sulfur-Rich Foods

FRIEND?

Foods that are naturally rich in sulfur are great immune boosters; support skin health; are antimicrobial; aid in microcirculation to joints, kidneys, eyes, and the heart; are essential for important detoxing processes; and they contribute to lowering blood pressure (if that is desired). We require sulfur to make proteins, and we need it for over a hundred physiological processes in the body. It is best to consume animal proteins and eggs with sulfur-rich amino acids *and* vegetables that are rich in organosulfur compounds. Both are important when living with Lyme.

Sulfur is needed for energy production in the cells and vital detoxification pathways in the liver. We need it for healthy joints, detox, and the production of glutathione, which is essential to the body's ability to get rid of heavy metals, cadmium, and aluminum. Two important sulfur-containing amino acids are cysteine and methionine. They are used in a biochemical process, called *methylation*, which affects how well our body can get rid of toxins, including metals such as cadmium and aluminum. We also need it for our heart health and to guard against strokes.[7] Individuals who favor a mostly plant-based diet run the risk of a sulfur deficiency, which will impact their ability to get rid of metals. This matters greatly with Lyme. (However, for detox, B vitamins and other minerals including magnesium and selenium are required.)

Protein-rich foods such as free-range meat, poultry, wild fish, eggs, nuts, and legumes are good dietary sources of sulfur. Eggs are rich in sulfur, especially the egg white.

Whole food plant sources, including the cruciferous family, are rich sources of sulfur-containing substances called *glucosinulates*. Chew these well to derive the full benefit. Other sources are asparagus, potatoes, okra, spinach, and squash.

Garlic, onions, leeks, and chives contain organosulfur compounds. These are antimicrobial; it is effective for yeast infections and cancers. In certain infections, and for certain individuals, high-dose garlic is part of a therapeutic regimen. Garlic also supports heart health as well as circulation in smaller blood vessels, and it is helpful in lowering elevated blood pressure.

FOE?

If you were allergic to sulfur, you would have never been born—it is that necessary! Some individuals do not tolerate sulfur-rich foods, and they experience digestive distress. There is a genetic component that can be in play, and mercury toxicity must also be considered.

Pyrrole, or pyroluria, is a biochemical challenge that is inherited or acquired with chronic infections such as Lyme and can induce intolerance of sulfur containing foods resulting in psychiatric symptoms. This condition was discovered in the 1950's by a Canadian research team led by Dr. Abram Hoffer. The body releases excessive amounts of zinc, vitamin B6, magnesium, and other nutrients that are needed for biochemical processes that involve sulfur. It is always about checks and balances in the body, as it is complex.

The sulfonamide molecule in antibiotics that many are allergic to contains sulfur, but it is that molecule—not sulfur itself—that causes reactions to sulfa drugs, sulfites, and sulfates.[8]

Sulfur-rich foods can create indigestion and other symptoms; garlic and onions can be contraindicated for some individuals. Often these individuals have a great dislike for garlic in any form, and they do their best to avoid it. Garlic can be hidden in salad dressings, oils, sauces, and spice mixes, especially in commercial foods and when eating out at restaurants.

Seaweed

FRIEND?

It is a great idea to include seaweed in your diet, such as nori, wakame, or miso in soups and stews. Minerals from seaweed will offset mineral deficiencies induced by consumption of the cruciferous vegetables. Seaweed is a great antidote to the thyroid inhibition from cruciferous vegetables (and soy). This is one reason why there is always seaweed in miso soup at a Japanese restaurants.

Iodine is deficient in the soil today, yet it is an important mineral for breast, ovarian, prostate, and thyroid health. The reproductive tissues all require iodine.

When dealing with chronic Lyme, the adrenals and thyroid are often challenged too, contributing to symptoms like fatigue, constipation, and moodiness. Zinc and selenium are the two minerals that must be present in adequate amounts to support iodine absorption and prevent a detox reaction. Whole foods contain their own mineral complexes, and adding seaweed into a pot of broth is an easy and nourishing addition. It is rich in minerals that we need, providing a good source of natural electrolyte support.

FOE?

With an autoimmune thyroid condition, such as Hashimoto's thyroiditis, restrict high iodine foods. Even though the thyroid needs nutrients (including iodine, zinc, selenium, and vitamin E), when antibodies are elevated, it is best to restrict additional iodine supplementation. It is important to know that breasts, ovaries, and prostates need iodine too.

A lot of the seaweed is contaminated because our rainwater and our oceans are contaminated. The meltdown of the nuclear reactor in Fukushima, Japan, had a great impact on thyroid health of children born on the Pacific coast after the meltdown. The meltdown also affected global seaweed and marine life. If possible, seek out products from the Atlantic Ocean. Sadly, we live in a very contaminated world, so check the sourcing of your foods as much as possible.

Wrapping Up

When living with Lyme, providing the body with an array of phytonutrients and bioflavoinoids is important. The key is to eliminate foods that irritate and add foods with a positive effect. Start by increasing the variety of foods you eat. Create a plate of food at mealtime that contains a protein, a healthy fat source, and two to three vegetables. At the end of the day, take note of how many different colored vegetables you ate that day or how many different oils you used that day. Gradually, become creative with your plate and your palate. Once a week, try a new food or a new way of preparing food; there are so many recipes online for all different dietary considerations.

If you have been diagnosed with SIBO or IBS/IBD and are on a low FOD-MAP diet already but you are not feeling better, perhaps you could add protein enzymes, ox bile, and hydrochloric acid into your program. Pay attention to your symptoms, and start to gradually and carefully increase the variety of your foods as best as you can. It must be done in small steps that you can manage, and the process is different for everyone. Do what feels right for you.

If secondary infections in the gut are cleared, the gut lining and adrenals are revitalized, and the microflora is more diverse, you will hopefully tolerate more and more foods over a period of time, whether you are in remission or active Lyme treatment. Healing is a lifelong process for each and everyone of us.

It is not easy to navigate through this difficult journey by yourself. The Lyme infection and coinfections can throw your eating habits and food choices for a loop during antibiotic treatment and herx reactions, and your symptoms can change on a dime. It is helpful to partner with a professional who can guide you nutritionally along the way, so you can focus on becoming well.

"If we had no hope—for a cure, for winning the lottery, for falling in love, for the end of war, for being free of abuse, or for having food, warmth, clothing, and shelter—we would have no reason to go on. What you hope for doesn't matter, but rather the essence of hope itself."

—BERNIE SIEGEL

Conclusion

Thank you for taking the time to read through this comprehensive book. At times, you might have thought that it was overwhelming. Perhaps you put the book down and waited a while before reading on—good. It takes time to process all this information, and it takes time to put it into action. At all times, you must choose your own path and pace; after all, it is not a race.

I admire the courage you bring to every single day of your life, with challenges that I cannot even imagine. Despite adversity, you are staying the course with self-education, tenacity, and mental toughness—against all odds, at times.

Many with Lyme-related illnesses are living a life of suffering, while trying to find a doctor who can help them with appropriate treatment. Some treatments are not tolerated and other treatment options must be explored. Mothers feel guilty because they unknowingly pass on infections to their children during pregnancy or while breastfeeding. Parents watch in despair as their babies, children, toddlers, and teenagers change before their eyes when infections take hold. I see parents who spare no expense to find the right treatment for their child. Bearing witness to the many lives filled with sickness, worry, disability, and devastation leaves me wanting to be of service in this community.

I also wish to honor those who have succumbed to these treacherous infections despite their best efforts. I implore you to keep seeking until you have found the right practitioners and doctors that will help you.

Despite adversity, it is individuals like you who will push this illness to the forefront and who will bring about change. There are many of you, and your courageous voice matters greatly.

At a recent Lyme conference, I was speaking to a distinguished retired surgeon from a top hospital in Massachusetts, who, with tears in his eyes, said that he wished he had known more about vector-borne infections and the labyrinth of persistent Lyme before his son became ill. His grown son had been in psychiatric treatment for three years. Many physicians misdiagnosed him, and the father wished he could have done more to help his son, but he did not know about these infections. Here he was, a top surgeon in his field, yet he was overwhelmed and distraught with tears in his eyes. It was a humbling moment to witness his despair and vulnerability. There are many, many stories like this, and many more stories that we do not hear about.

Where Are We Now?

IN THE UNITED STATES

It is encouraging that there is more interest in chronic Lyme and its coinfections from major institutions in the United States today, including the research by Dr. Ying Zhang at John Hopkins, scientific studies by Dr. Kim Lewis from Northeastern, and new research in tick-borne infections at the Mayo Clinic.

Senator Blumenthal has been an outspoken proponent by asking for more government funds to improve current archaic laboratory blood testing, better reporting of tick-borne infections, and reintroduced the Lyme and Tick-Borne Disease Protection Education and Research Act, which is intended to increase awareness and education in the medical community.[1]

In Rhode Island, Sen. Jack Reed secured 23 million dollars in Lyme disease research grants.

Governor Andrew Cuomo in New York State signed a bill that gives more protection to physicians who prescribed prolonged antibiotics for Lyme disease under state law. This is a big step in a hard-won battle, and it was received with great joy by the medical-literate Lyme community.

In Massachusetts, the state House of Representatives and the Senate reenacted the Lyme legislation that requires insurers in the state to cover Lyme disease treatment for as long as a doctor says it would benefit the ill patient. Governor Charlie Baker vetoed the bill, which was supported by over five hundred infectious disease doctors and insurance companies. I am thrilled to write that the veto was overturned by decisive action from the House and Senate. The House voted 153 to 3, and the Senate voted 37 to 1, a great victory for physicians and patients in Massachusetts and all in the Lyme community.

The Virginia senate passed a new Lyme disease bill in its commitment to taking the threat of Lyme disease very seriously. The recommended guidelines from the Infectious Disease Society of America (IDSA) are considered outdated.[2]

On another positive note, the IDSA treatment guidelines and protocols have been removed from the website of the National Guideline Clearinghouse (NGC). The NGC is an initiative of the Agency for Healthcare Research and Quality, United States Department of Health and Human Services, which is used as a reference for physicians and healthcare practitioners in treating patients.

However, many doctors are hesitant in treating Lyme or vector-borne illness for the long term because of sanctions from their state medical boards. It still is a "political football," and this holds true for many states. The complaints to medical boards are lodged by insurance companies, not patients. . . .

Existing research has not sufficiently extended into the multiple coinfection strains that occur on a global scale, and lack of funding for research is another challenge. The immense diversity of strains makes these infections difficult to test, diagnose, and treat, and there is great variance in treatment approaches. Germany, Austria, France, Norway, Czech Republic, Slovenia, Slovakia, Belgium, Finland, Japan, Switzerland, Sweden, and China are acknowledging the endemic existence of these infections, yet appropriate diagnoses and treatment is lacking for many who are seriously ill.[3]

Official reportings and real incidences differ greatly. Few countries have made these infections mandatorily notifiable, and this makes it difficult to track data, especially with underreporting and non-standardarized testing of coinfections. Currently, there is no European consensus on antibiotic treatment in acute or long-term vector-borne infections. Antibiotic resistance concerns and not enough scientific data to support the efficacy of prolonged treatment are common arguing points.

For more information on specialized testing options, see the resources section at the back of the book. For more guidance on Lyme-treating health professionals and physicians, check the resources online at ILADS.org. Lyme-Literate Medical Doctors (LLMDs), patients, families, Lyme advocacy groups, and concerned citizens constantly challenge inadequate current CDC treatment guidelines, the nonsupportive medical establishment, and insurance companies. That is a tall order for those in the Lyme battlefield.

Research on a global scale is ongoing and new tests are being developed, but this is still happening within a vacuum of special interest groups and profit-driven medical and political wrangling, as was recently witnessed in Massachusetts.

· · · · · · ·

Wrapping Up

I am also very grateful for those physicians who show interest and a willingness to learn about all that is encompassed in Lyme and toxic mold–related infections, even if they are not specialists in that area. We must keep learning; after all, we are students of life. It is those forward-thinking doctors, who are on your side and want you to be better, that support your healing path. When I met Dr. Jeffrey Bland at the Functional Forum in New York City, I mentioned to him that we must address persistent Lyme-related infections in the functional medicine paradigm. He agreed and told me to "keep the conversation going"—and that is what I am doing, every day.

As a practitioner, I am honored to be part of the integrative and forward-thinking Lyme community that is willing to push boundaries and to serve their patients of any age. I am grateful and thankful for the support of those who push the frontiers of cutting-edge science in the world. These physicians are not afraid to take on commercial paradigms; to the contrary, they apply an open mind, uncommercial treatment, nutritional therapies, and alternative modalities in their patient-centered treatment—and not with financial gains in mind. They treat incredibly difficult cases over many years, and they restore lives and hope to many.

It is with gratitude that I support the individuals who see me in my private practice. I do not have all the answers, not by a long shot; but in every case, I will pursue all options that can help my patient improve the quality of their life. I am not a physician, but it does not mean that I cannot strive to make a difference; and it does not mean that I cannot collaborate with esteemed physicians in this field. I will not walk away from one of the greatest health challenges we are currently faced with.

Together we can make a difference; together we can bring about change. By collaborating from a place of integrity, authenticity, and from a place in the heart and soul, we can bring about meaningful change that will affect many lives today and in the years to come. May you stay on your chosen wellness path with courage, resilience, and hope.

To you, the reader—

I salute you.

May you nourish, heal, and thrive.

An Easy and Practical Shopping List

In the cabinet

- Organic coconut or palm oil
- Cold-pressed olive oil
- Unrefined sunflower and evening primrose oil
- Raw cacao
- Quinoa or rice if tolerated
- Coconut or almond flour
- Rice
- Gelatin options include Great Lakes, vital proteins, or Bulletproof
- Legumes, whole or canned BPA-free lining
- Herbal Teas
- Raw local honey
- Aluminum-free baking powder
- Organic tomato sauce
- A fiber supplement
- Stevia leaf (optional)

Food choices for quick meal preparation (in BP-free lined cans)

- Coconut milk
- Black beans
- Wild salmon
- Wild sardines in water

In the spice rack

- Sea salt
- Black pepper
- Turmeric
- Cumin
- Cinnamon
- Dried herbs
- Seaweed flakes
- Bay leaves

In the freezer

- Pasture-raised animal meats
- Free-range chicken
- Marrow bones
- Wild fish
- Organic butter
- Organ meats
- Organic Vegetables
- Berries

In the fridge

- Cod liver oil
- Tahini or hummus
- Evening primrose oil
- Olives

- Seed butter
- Fermented vegetables and/or pickles (if tolerated)
- Raw apple cider vinegar
- Organic butter or ghee
- Fermented foods
- Whole flaxseeds
- Organic produce
- Chia seeds
- Non-denatured protein powder
- Unsweetened apple sauce

Shopping Tips

PRODUCE

Choose fresh, ripe, in season, and locally grown produce from the farmer's market or a food co-op. Choose multiple colors, each one has its own antioxidants and vitamins.

MEATS AND POULTRY

Choose pasture raised, antibiotic-free, and hormone-free meats and poultry. And be sure that they were not fed with food containing soy or corn. Butcher cuts are safer than ground meats. If possible, have your butcher grind a whole cut for you. If possible, avoid frozen poultry unless you get it from the farmer or market.

SEAFOOD

Choose smaller fish from cold water, nonfarm-raised fish or seafood. Sadly, all fish by now are contaminated with environmental pollutants and toxins. Fish should smell like the sea and the eyes of the fish must be clear, not cloudy. Consider consumption of additional nutrients to protect against heavy metal exposure. Avoid raw fish consumption (risk of parasites).

HERBS

If possible, grow your herbs in a pot. If not, purchase dried herbs, which are more concentrated than fresh herbs.

LABELS

Check expiration dates and check labels; the fewer ingredients listed on a label, the better. Check for a whole food description on the label and look at the sugars listed.

Rika's Simply Nutritious Shakes

Please consider all food sensitivities, food allergies, and digestive limitations before consuming any of these shakes. Use purified water only. Keep in mind that leftover steamed vegetables are a great addition to any shake. Be creative! (Caution: Stevia can affect biofilm and Lyme, so a little raw honey might be a better option at this time.) Simply add the ingredients for each shake to a blender, mix, and enjoy.

Savory Broth Shake

- 1 ½ cups of chicken or bone both
- 1 tablespoon of whole flaxseeds
- 1 cup of steamed kale, one cup of cooked cabbage, or one cup of cooked lentils
- 1 ½ tablespoons of almond butter or coconut oil
- A sprinkle of turmeric and sea salt (black pepper optional)

Coco-Choco Shake

- 1 cup of unsweetened almond or coconut milk
- ½ to ¼ cup of water
- 2 scoops of a high-quality protein powder.
- 1 cup of steamed kale
- 1 cup of berries or ½ cup of pomegranate
- 1 teaspoon or MCT oil or flaxseed oil OR
- 1 tablespoon whole flaxseeds
- 1 teaspoon of raw cacao
- Sprinkle of cinnamon (optional)
- Stevia (optional)

Green Banana Shake

- 1 ½ ounces of water
- 2 scoops of protein powder or a serving of gelatin powder
- 1 teaspoon of unrefined safflower oil or sunflower oil
- ½ less-ripe banana
- 1 teaspoon of pomegranate powder
- 1 handful of steamed kale
- Sprinkle of sea salt

Cocoberry Dessert Shake

- 1 cup of unsweetened coconut milk
- ½ cup water
- 1 cup of mixed frozen berries (bring to room temperature)
- 1 scoop of spirulina or organic mixed greens
- 1 teaspoon of hempseed oil or evening primrose oil
- 1 tablespoon of raw cacao or cacao nips
- Stevia (optional)

Appendix C

Rika's Favorite Bone Marrow Broth

Broth makes a great base for any vegetable soup, stew or sauce. With chronic Lyme, chronic fatigue, and any digestive troubles, broth is a part of a nourishing eating strategy. Yes, it takes planning and some work, but in the end, it's worth it. I recommend beginning with this recipe. You are welcome to add herbs and spices according to what you like and can tolerate.

Getting Ready

- Defrost 2 pounds of frozen marrowbones (unless you have fresh bones from the butcher or farmer).
- Place the marrowbones in a stockpot, Crock-Pot, or a pot with higher sides and a lid.
- Fill up the pot with water until the bones are well covered.
- Add 1 teaspoon of sea salt or add sea vegetables.
- Add 3 tablespoons of raw apple cider vinegar.

Let's Get Cookin'

- Place the pot on the stovetop and bring the bones in water to a boil. (You want to be in the kitchen to prevent any accidental overflow.)
- Turn down to a simmer and cover (leave a slight opening for steam to evaporate).
- Intermittently, skim off any brown foam from the top of the bones.

Keep the bones simmering for roughly four hours. (Chicken, turkey, and fish bones and skin need roughly two hours.) It depends on the amount of bones, the size of the pot, and the temperature you are cooking with. Use these instructions as a general guideline and fine-tune it to your needs.

Check on the broth regularly and skim off more foam when needed, and should too much water have evaporated, add more. You want the bones to be covered at all times to support the release of minerals and cartilage from the bones, which creates the delicious and nutritious gelatin.

When using seaweed, it can get stuck in the foam. Separate it and keep it in the pot for mineral extraction.

After four hours, carefully take the bones out of the pot and place them in a separate container. Be careful; they are very hot. Then grab your mittens, hold the pot, and pour all liquid through a sieve into a holding container, ideally a porcelain dish with a glass lid. Caution—the liquid is hot! It is best if you get someone to help you hold the sieve while the other person pours out the broth or stock.

You can also turn off the stove to allow the stock to cool down a little before taking out the bones and pouring the broth through a sieve. See what works best for you.

Should you have too much liquid, reduce the liquid by keeping the pot on the stovetop for another thirty to sixty minutes; otherwise, you will have a runny broth. It is still nutritious in a diluted form, but it is, and tastes, watery.

Allow the broth to cool or indulge in a cup. Season the broth according to your taste or tolerance. It is now ready to be enjoyed.

Once the bones cool down, you can peel off additional gelatin (cartilage) that might still be on the bones. This is a great source of bioavailable protein.

Bone marrow is a rich, nourishing traditional food. If tolerated, add a sprinkle of sea salt and eat a small portion of bone marrow as part of a meal. A little goes a long way. It is very rich in nourishing cholesterol.

Once the broth has cooled, place it in the refrigerator, and let it cool overnight.

The next morning, you can skim the white fat layer off the broth. This is especially helpful if you do not tolerate heavy (saturated) fats well. The broth should be gelatinous, with a "sloppy" consistency.

Enjoy a cup of nourishing broth or add in some steamed vegetables and enjoy a hearty vegetable soup for your next meal.

Leftover broth can be stored in mason jars in the freezer. (Leave a good bit of room in the top of the jar so that it doesn't explode.)

Endnotes

Introduction

1.   Michael J. Cook, "Lyme Borrelliosis: A Review of Data on Transmission Time After Tick Attachment," *International Journal of General Medicine* 8 (2015): 1–8, doi: 10.2147/IJGM.S73791.

2.   Lyme Disease Research Database, "Alan MacDonald Interview," Lyme Disease Research Database (2005) www.lyme-disease-research-database.com/alan-macdonald-transcription.html

3.   Gary P. Wormser, Raymond J. Dattwyler, Eugene D. Shapiro, John J. Halperin, Allen C. Steere, Mark S. Klempner, Peter J. Krause, Johan S. Bakken, Franc Strle, Gerold Stanek, Linda Bockenstedt, Durland Fish, J. Stephen Dumler, and Robert B. Nadelman, "The Clinical Assessment, Treatment, and Prevention of Lyme Disease, Human Granulocytic Anaplasmosis, and Babesiosis: Clinical Practice Guidelines by the Infectious Diseases Society of America," *Clinical Infectious Diseases* 43, no. 9 (2006): 1089–1134, doi: 10.1086/508667.

4.   Muqing Li, Toshiyuki Masuzawa, Nobuhiro Takada, Fubito Ishiguro, Hiromi Fujita, Atsue Iwaki, Haipeng Wang, Juchun Wang, Masato Kawabata, and Yasutake Yanagihara, "Lyme Disease *Borrelia* Species in Northeastern China Resemble Those Isolated from Far Eastern Russia and Japan," *Applied and Environmental Microbiology* 64, no. 7 (1998): 2705–2709.

5. Centers for Disease Control and Prevention, "Preliminary Maps and Data for 2015," Centers for Disease Control and Prevention (Atlanta, 2005) http://www.cdc.gov/westnile/statsmaps/preliminarymapsdata/index.html

6. Jason Tan, Christine H. Smith, and Ran D. Goldman, "Pediatric Autoimmune Neuropsychiatric Disorders Associated with Streptococcal Infections," *Canadian Family Physician* 58, no. 9 (2012): 957–959.

7. Thamotharampillai Dileepan, Erica D. Smith, Daniel Knowland, Martin Hsu, Maryann Platt, Peter Bittner-Eddy, Brenda Cohen, Peter Southern, Elizabeth Latimer, Earl Harley, Dritan Agalliu, and P. Patrick Cleary, "Group A *Streptococcus* Intranasal Infection Promotes CNS Infiltration by Streptococcal-Specific Th17 Cells," *The Journal of Clinical Investigation* 126, no. 1 (2016): 303–317.

Chapter Two

1. Howard F. Jenkinson and L. Julia Douglas, "Interactions Between *Candida* Species and Bacteria in Mixed Infections," in *Polymicrobial Diseases*, ed. Kim A. Brogden and Janet M. Guthmiller (Washington, DC: American Society of Microbiology Press, 2002).

2. Carlos Magno da Costa Maranduba, Sandra Bertelli Ribeiro De Castro, Gustavo Torres de Souza, Cristiano Rossato, Francisco Carlos da Guia, Maria Anete Santana Valente, Joao Vitor Paes Rettore, Claudineia Pereira Maranduba, Camila Maurmann de Souza, Antonio Marcio Resende do Carmo, Gilson Costa Macedo, and Fernando de Sá Silva, "Intestinal Microbiota as Modulators of the Immune System and Neuroimmune System: Impact on the Host Health and Homeostasis," *Journal of Immunology Research* (2015), doi: 10.1155/2015/931574.

3. Amy Langdon, Nathan Crook, and Gautam Dantas, "The Effects of Antibiotics on the Microbiome Throughout Development and Alternative Approaches for Therapeutic Modulation," *Genome Medicine* 8, no. 1 (2016): 39, doi: 10.1186/s13073-016-0294-z.

4.	D. Berg, L. H. Berg, J. Couvaras, and H. Harrison, "Chronic Fatigue Syndrome and/or Fibromyalgia as a Variation of Antiphospholipid Antibody Syndrome: An Explanatory Model and Approach to Laboratory Diagnosis," *Blood Coagulation and Fibrinolysis* 10, no. 7 (1999): 435–8.

5.	Allen C. Steere, Jenifer Coburn, and Lisa Glickstein, "The Emergence of Lyme Disease," *The Journal of Clinical Investigation* 113, no. 8 (2004): 1093–1101, doi: 10.1172/JCI200421681.

6.	A. B. Csoka, M. Szyf, "Epigenetic Side-Effects of Common Pharmaceuticals: A Potential New Field in Medicine and Pharmacology," *Medical Hypotheses* 73, no. 5 (2008): 770–80, doi: 10.1016/j.mehy2008.10.039.

7.	"LDN and HIV/AIDS," Low Dose Naltrexone, http://www.lowdosenaltrexone.org/ldn_and_hiv.htm

8.	"LDN and Multiple Sclerosis (MS)," Low Dose Naltrexone, http://www.lowdosenaltrexone.org/ldn_and_ms.htm

9.	C. K. Ong, P. Lirk, C. H. Tan, and R. A. Seymour, "An Evidence-Based Update on Nonsteroidal Anti-Inflammatory Drugs," *Clinical Medical Research* 5, no. 1 (2007): 19–34, doi: 10.3121/cmr.2007.698.

10.	Nagaraja Moorthy, N. Raghavendra, P. N. Venkatarathnamma, "Levofloxacin-Induced Acute Psychosis," *Indian Journal of Psychiatry* 50, no. 1 (2008): 57–58, doi: 10.4103/0019-5545.39762.

11.	"How Sleep Clears the Brain," National Institutes of Health, NIH Research Matters, last modified October 28, 2013, https://www.nih.gov/news-events/nih-research-matters/how-sleep-clears-brain

12.	Janet K. Kern, David A. Geier, Tapan Audhya, Paul G. King, Lisa K. Sykes, and Mark R. Geier, "Evidence of Parallels between Mercury Intoxication and the Brain Pathology in Autism," *Acta Neurobiologiae Experimentalis* 72, no. 2 (2012): 113–153, http://www.ncbi.nlm.nih.gov/pubmed/22810216

13.	"Conclusions," BioIntiative 2012, http://www.bioinitiative.org/conclusions/

Chapter Three

1. "GM Crops Now Banned in 38 Countries Worldwide—Sustainable Pulse Research," Sustainable Pulse, last modified October 22, 2015, http://sustainablepulse.com/2015/10/22/gm-crops-now-banned-in-36-countries-worldwide-sustainable-pulse-research/#.V1gyQ1eNQlI

2. Alberto Finamore, Marianna Roselli, Serena Britti, Giovanni Monastra, Roberto Ambra, Aida Turrini, and Elena Mengheri, "Intestinal and Peripheral Immune Response to MON810 Maize Ingestion in Weaning and Old Mice," *Journal of Agricultural and Food Chemistry* 56, no. 23 (2008): 11533–11539, doi: 10.1021/jf802059w.

3. Samuel S. Epstein, "Unlabeled Milk from Cows Treated with Biosynthetic Growth Hormones: A Case of Regulatory Abdication," *International Journal of Health Services* 20, no. 1 (1996): 173–185, doi: 10.2190/EDK8-T5RC-LUMR-B2H7.

4. Siriporn Thongprakaisang, Apinya Thiantanawat, Nuchanart Rangkadilok, Tawit Suriyo, and Jutamaad Satayavivad, "Glyphosate induces Human Breast Cancer Cells Growth via Estrogen Receptors," *Food and Chemical Toxicology* 59 (2013): 129–136, doi: 10.1016/j.fct.2013.05.057.

5. Anthony Samsel and Stephanie Seneff, "Glyphosate, Pathways to Modern Diseases III: Manganese, Neurological Diseases, and Associated Pathologies," *Surgical Neurology International* 6 (2015): 45, doi: 10.4103/2152-7806.153876.

6. Anthony Samsel and Stephanie Seneff, "Glyphosate, Pathways to Modern Diseases II: Celiac Sprue and Gluten Intolerance," *Interdisciplinary Toxicology* 6, no. 4 (2013): 159–184, doi: 10.2478/intox-2013-0026.

7. Artemis Dona and Ioannis Arvanitoyannis, "Health Risks of Genetically Modified Foods," *Critical Reviews in Food Science and Nutrition* 49, no. 2 (2009): 164–175, doi: 10.1080/10408390701855993.

8.   Imran Patanwala, Maria J. King, David A. Barrett, John Rose, Ralph Jackson, Mark Hudson, Mark Philo, Jack R. Dainty, Anthony J. A. Wright, Paul M. Finglas, and David E. Jones, "Folic Acid Handling by the Human Gut: Implications for Food Fortification and Supplementation," *The American Journal of Clinical Nutrition* 100, no. 2 (2014): 593–588, doi: 10.3945/ajcn.113.080507.

9.   Young-In Kim, "Does a High Folate Intake Increase the Risk of Breast Cancer?" *Nutrition Reviews* 64, no. 10 (2006): 468–475, doi: 10.1111/j.1753-4887.2006.tb00178.x.

Chapter Four

1.   Roberto Berni Canani, Margherita Di Costanzo, Ludovica Leone, Monica Pedata, Rosaria Meli, and Antonio Calignano, "Potential Beneficial Effects of Butyrate in Intestinal and Extraintestinal Diseases," *World Journal of Gastroenterology* 17, no. 12 (2011): 1519–1528, doi: 10.3748/wjg.v17.i12.1519.

2.   Jessica R. Jackson, William W. Eaton, Nicola G. Cascella, Alessio Fasano, and Deanna L. Kelley, "Neurologic and Psychiatric Manifestations of Celiac Disease and Gluten Sensitivity," *Psychiatric Quarterly* 83, no. 1 (2012): 91–102, doi: 10.1007/s11126-011-9186-y.

3.   Joseph V. Campellone, "Migraine," *Medline Plus*, last modified January 5, 2016, https://medlineplus.gov/ency/article/000709.htm

4.   Jim Core, "Study Examines Long-Term Health Effects of Soy Infant Formula," *Agricultural Research* 52, no. 1 (2004), https://agresearchmag.ars.usda.gov/2004/jan/soy

5.   Jameson T. Crowley, Alvaro M. Toledo, Timothy J. LaRocca, James L. Coleman, Erwin London, and Jorge L. Benach, "Lipid Exchange between *Borrelia burgdorferi* and Host Cells," *PloS Pathogens* 9, no. 1 (2013), doi: 10.1371/journal.ppat.1003109.

6.   David S. Cassarino and James P. Bennett, Jr, "An Evaluation of the role of Mitochondria in Neurodegenerative Diseases: Mitochondrial Mutations and Oxidative Pathology, Protective Nuclear Responses, and

Cell Death in Neurodegeneration," *Brain Research Reviews* 29, no. 1 (1999): 1–25, http://www.ncbi.nlm.nih.gov/pubmed/9974149

7. Patty W. Siri-Tarino, Qi Sun, Frank B. Hu, and Ronald M. Krauss, "Meta-Analysis of Prospective Cohort Studies Evaluating the Association of Saturated Fat with Cardiovascular Disease," *The American Journal of Clinical Nutrition* 91, no. 3 (2010): 535–546, doi: 10.3945/ajcn.2009.2772.

8. T. A. Manolio, W. H. Ettinger, R. P. Tracy, L. H. Kuller, N. O. Borhani, J. C. Lynch, and L. P. Fried, "Epidemiology of Low Cholesterol Levels in Older Adults. The Cardiovasculary Health Study," *Circulation* 87, no. 3 (1993): 728–737, doi: 10.1161/01.CIR.87.3.728.

9. Annie L. Culver, Ira S. Ockene, Raji Balasubramanian, Barbara C. Olendzki, Deidre M. Sepavich, Jean Wactawski-Wende, JoAnn E. Manson, Yongxia Qiao, Simin Liu, Philip A. Merriam, Catherine Rahilly-Tierny, Fridtjof Thomas, Jeffrey S. Berger, Judith K. Ockene, J. David Curb, and Yunsheng Ma, "Statin Use and Risk of Diabetes Mellitus in Postmenopausal Women in the Women's Health Initiative," *JAMA Internal Medicine* 172, no. 2 (2012): 144–152, doi: 10.1001/archinternmed.2011.625.

10. Guy D. Eslick, Peter R. C. Howe, Caroline Smith, Ros Priest, and Alan Bensoussan, "Benefits of Fish Oil Supplementation in Hyperlipidemia: A Systematic Review and Meta-analysis," *International Journal of Cardiology* 136, no. 1 (2009): 4–16, doi: 10.1016/j.ijcard.2008.03.092.

11. L. A. Horrocks and Y. K. Yeo, "Health Benefits of Docosahexaenoic Acid (DHA)," *Pharmacological Research* 40, no. 3 (1999): 211–225, http://www.ncbi.nlm.nih.gov/pubmed/10479465

12. Susan R. Sturgeon, Joanna L. Heersink, Stella L. Volpe, Elizabeth R. Bertone-Johnson, Elaine Puleo, Frank Z. Stanczyk, Sara Sabelawski, Kristina Wähälä, Mindy S. Kurzer, and Carol Bigelow, "Effect of Dietary Flaxseed on Serum Levels of Estrogens and Androgens in Postmenopausal Women," *Nutrition and Cancer* 60, no. 5 (2008): 612–618, doi: 10.1080/01635580801971864.

13. Debra A. Nowak, Denise C. Snyder, Ann J. Brown, and Wendy
     Demark-Wahnefried, "The Effect of Flaxseed supplementation on
     Hormonal Levels Associated with Polcystic Ovarian Syndrome: A Case
     Study," *Current Topics in Nutraceutical Research* 5, no. 4: 177–181, http://
     www.ncbi.nlm.nih.gov/pmc/articles/PMC2752973

Chapter Five

1.   Magda Havas, "Dirty Electricity Elevates Blood Sugar Among
     Eletrically Sensitive Diabetics and May Explain Brittle Diabetes,"
     Electromagnetic Biology and Medicine 27, no. 2 (2008): 135–146, doi:
     10.1080/15368370802072075.

4   Scott A. Kinlein, Christopher D. Wilson, and Ilia N. Karatsoreos, "Dys-
     regulate Hypothalamic-Pituitary-Adrenal Axis Function Contributes to
     Altered Endocrine and Neurobehavioral Responses to Acute Stress,"
     Frontiers in Psychiatry 6, no. 31, doi: 10.3389/fpsyt.2015.00031.

5   Evanthia Diamanti-Kandarakis, Jean-Pierre Bourguignon, Linda C.
     Guidice, Russ Hauser, Gail S. Prins, Ana M. Soto, R. Thomas Zoeller,
     and Andrea C. Gore, "Endocrine-Disrupting Chemicals: An Endo-
     crine Society Scientific Statement," *Endocrine Review* 30, no. 4 (2009):
     293–342, doi: 10.1210/er.2009-0002.

6   Iain Scott, "The Role of Mitochondria in the Mammalian Antivi-
     ral Defense System," *Mitochondrion* 10, no. 4 (2010): 316–320, doi:
     10.1016/j.mito.2010.02.005.

7   Sameer Kalghatgi, Catherine S. Spina, James C. Costello, Marc Liesa,
     J. Ruben Morones-Ramirez, Shimyn Slomovic, Anthony Molina, Orian
     S. Shirihai, and James J. Collins, "Bactericidal Antibiotics Induce
     Mitochondrial Dysfunction and Oxidative Damage in Mammalian
     Cells," *Science Translational Medicine* 5, no. 192: 192ra85, doi: 10.1126/
     scitranslmed.3006055.

Chapter Six

1. "Xylitol as a Sweetener and Biofilm Buster," MD Junction Online Support Group, Lyme Disease, 2013, http://www. mdjunction.com/forums/lyme-disease-support-forums/ general-support/10797675-xylitol-as-a-sweetener-and-biofilm-buster

Chapter Seven

1. James M. Ferguson, "SSRI Antidepressant Medications: Adverse Effects and Tolerability," *Primary Care Companion to the Journal of Clinical Psychiatry* 3, no. 1 (2001): 22-27, http://www.ncbi.nlm.nih.gov/ pmc/articles/PMC181155/

2. Philip A. Mackowiak, "Recycling Metchnikoff: Probiotics, the Intestinal Microbiome, and the Quest for Long Life," *Frontiers in Public Health* 1, (2013): 52, doi: 10.3389/fpubh.2013.00052.

3. S. P. Stabler and R. H. Allen, "Vitamin B12 Deficiency as a Worldwide Problem," *Annual Review of Nutrition* 24 (2004): 299–326, doi: 10.1146/annurev.nutr.24.012003.132440.

4. Perlmutter, David, "Gluten Associated Cross Reactive Foods," http:// www.drperlmutter.com/eat/foods-that-cross-react-with-gluten/

5. National Institute of Health, "Autoimmune Diseases Coordinating Committee: Autoimmune Diseases Research Plan," US Department of Health and Human Services (2005).

6. Abner Louis Notkins, "New Predictors of Disease," *Scientific American* 296 (2007): 72–79, doi: 10.1038/scientificamerican0307-72.

7. Caitriona M. Guinane, Amany Tadrousc, Fiona Fouhy, C. Anthony Ryan, Eugene M. Dempsey, Brendan Murphy, Emmet Andrewsc, Paul D. Cotter, Catherine Stanton, and R. Paul Ross, "Microbial Composition of Human Appendices from Patients Following Appendectomy," *mBio* 4, no. 1 (2013), doi: 10.1128/mBio.00366-12.

Chapter Eight

1. Enzo Ierardi, Claudia Sorrentino, Mariabeatrice Principi, Floriana Giorgio, Giuseppe Losurdo, and Alfredo Di Leo, "Intestinal Microbial Metabolism of Phosphatidylcholine: A Novel Insight in the Cardiovascular Risk Scenario," *Hepatobiliary Surgery and Nutrition* 4, no. 4 (2015): 289–292, doi: 10.3978/j.issn.2304-3881.2015.02.01.

Chapter Nine

1. Andrew C. Dukowicz, Brian E. Lacy, and Gary M. Levine, "Small Intestinal Bacterial Overgrowth," *Gastroenterology and Hepatology* 3, no. 2 (2007): 112–122, http://www.ncbi.nlm.nih.gov/pmc/articles/PMC3099351/

Chapter Eleven

1. Sarah R. Brand, Stephanie M. Engel, Richard L. Canfield, and Rachel Yehuda, "The Effect of Maternal PTSD Following In Utero Trauma Exposure on Behavior and Temperament in the 9-Month-Old Infant," *Annals of the New York Academy of Sciences* 1071 (2006): 454–8, doi: 10.1196/annals.1364.041.

2. Rachel Yehuda, Martin H. Teicher, Jonathan R. Secki, Robert A. Grossman, Adam Morris, and Linda M. Bierer, "Parental Posttraumatic Stress Disorder as a Vulnerability Factor for Low Cortisol Trait in Offspring of Holocaust Survivors," *Archives of General Psychiatry* 64, no.9 (2007): 1040–8, doi: 10.1001/archpsyc.64.9.1040.

Chapter Twelve

1. Jessica R. Jackson, William W. Eaton, Nicola G. Cascella, Alessio Fasano, and Deanna L. Kelly, "Neurologic and Psychiatric Manifestations of Celiac Disease and Gluten Sensitivity," *Psychiatric Quarterly* 83, no. 1 (2012): 91–102, doi: 10.1007/s11126-011-9186-y.

2. Andrew C. Dukowicz, Brian E. Lacy, and Gary M. Levine, "Small Intestinal Bacterial Overgrowth," *Gastroenterology and Hepatology* 3, no. 2 (2007): 112–122, http://www.ncbi.nlm.nih.gov/pmc/articles/PMC3099351/

3. Rana S. Bonds and Terumi Midoro-Horiuti, "Estrogen Effects in Allergy and Asthma," *Current Opinion in Allergy and Clinical Immunology* 13, no. 1 (2013): 92–99, doi: 10.1097/ACI.0b013e32835a6dd6.

4. Bruna Guida, C. D. De Martino, S. D. De Martino, Giovanni Tritto, Vicenzo Patella, R. Trio, C. D'Agostino, P. Pecoraro, and Luciano D'Agostino, "Histamine Plasma Levels and Elimination Diet in Chronic Idiopathic Urticaria," *European Journal of Clinical Nutrition* 54, no. 2 (2000): 155–158, doi: 10.1038/sj.ejcn.1600911.

5. Kan Shida, Tadashi Sato, Ryoko Iizuka, Ryotaro Hoshi, Osamu Watanabe, Tomoki Igarashi, Kouji Miyazaki, Masanobu Nanno, and Fumiyasu Ishikawa, "Daily Intake of Fermented Milk with *Lactobacillus casei* Strain Shirota Reduces the Incidence and Duration of Upper Respiratory Tract Infections in Healthy Middle-Aged Office Workers," *European Journal of Nutrition* (2015), doi: 10.1007/s00394-015-1056-1.

6. Stephan C. Bischoff, Giovanni Barbara, Wim Buurman, Theo Ockhuizen, Jörg-Dieter Schulzke, Matteo Serino, Herbert Tilg, Alastair Watson, and Jerry M. Wells, "Intestinal Permeability – A New Target for Disease Prevention and Therapy," *BMC Gastroenterology* 14: 189, doi: 10.1186/s12876-014-0189-7.

7. Yves Ingenbleek and Hideo Kimura, "Nutritional Essentiality of Sulfur in Health and Disease," *Nutrition Review* 71, no. 7 (2013): 413–432, doi: 10.1111/nure.12050.

8. Edward Zimmer, "Allergic to Sulfa Drugs: Can You Take Sulfur?" Zimmer Nutrition, https://www.zimmernutrition.com/learning-center/health-articles/article/allergic-to-sulfa-drugs-can-you-take-sulfur/

Conclusion

1. Rebecca Shabad, "Dem Senator Wants More Funds to Research Lyme Disease," *The Hill*, June 8, 2015, http://thehill.com/policy/finance/244278-dem-senator-calls-for-additional-funding-to-research-lyme-disease

2. David Michael Conner, "A Big Week for Lyme Disease Patient and Physician Rights," *Huffington Post*, February 2, 2016, http://www.huffingtonpost.com/david-michael-conner/a-big-week-for-lyme-disea_b_9230980.html

3. Xian-Bo Wu, Ren-Hua Na, Shan-Shan Wei, Jin-Song Zhu, and Hong-Juan Peng, "Distribution of Tick-Borne Diseases in China," *Parasites & Vectors* 6 (2013): 119, doi: 10.1186/1756-3305-6-119.

Resources

Lyme and Biotoxin Resources

http://ilads.org

https://www.lymedisease.org

https://forumforintegrativemedicine.org

https://www.aaemonline.org (American Academy of Environmental Medicine)

http://www.klinghardtacademy.com

http://www.lymeresearchalliance.org

https://www.facebook.com/drrichardhorowitz/?fref=ts

http://www.prohealth.com/lyme/lyme-disease-organizations.cfm

http://lymediseasechallenge.org/financial-assistance/

http://www.survivingmold.com

http://www.westonaprice.org/dentistry/

http://www.ilads.org/media/boston/videos/videos_corson.php

http://www.ilads.org/media/washingtondc/videos/videos-Joseph_G_Jemsek_MD.php

http://www.cangetbetter.com

http://danielcameronmd.com/daniel-cameron-md-lyme-blog/

https://www.youtube.com/watch?v=THZhANfFnyY (Dr. Klinghardt / Pyyrole)

http://lisanagy.com

http://www.tiredoflyme.com/horowitz-lyme-msids-questionnaire.html

https://www.youtube.com/watch?v=r8tESJVvM88 (Dr. Alan MacDonald)

Specialized Lab Testing for Lyme and Coinfections

DNAConnexions

IGeneX, Inc.

Advanced Laboratory Services

Fry Clinical Laboratories

Stonybrook

Arminlabs (Europe)

Limbach Group SE (Europe)

Lyme DOT-BLOT

Galaxy Diagnostics

Medical Diagnostic Laboratories

Nanotrap Lyme Antigen test

Lyme Disease International Resources

Canadian Lyme Disease Foundation

Lyme Disease Action (United Kingdom)

Lyme Disease Association of Australia

Karl McManus Foundation (Australia)

France Lyme

Tick Talk Ireland

Lyme Poland

Deutsche Lyme Borreliose Hilfe

Association Luxembourgeoise Borréliose de Lyme (Luxembourg)

NorVect (Norway)

Biotoxin Testing

ERMI testing: https://www.emlab.com/s/services/ERMI_testing.html

Visual Acuity Test: http://www.survivingmold.com/diagnosis/visual-contrast-sensitivity-vcs

HLA DR / C3a / C4a / MSH/ in blood test

Diagnostic Laboratory Medicine: Nasal culture testing

Remediation: http://www.survivingmold.com/legal-resources/environmental/all-resources

Australia: http://www.survivingmold.com/treatment/surviving-mold-down-under

Testing and lab kits are available from P&K Microbiology, or you can use an environmental mold index test.

Functional Medicine and Functional Nutrition Labs

BioHealth Laboratory

Great Plains Laboratory

Diagnostic Solutions Laboratory (GI MAP test)

DRG Laboratory

EnteroLab

Commonwealth Labs

Oxford Biomedical: Mediator Release Test (MRT)

Genova Diagnostics

Doctor's Data

Cyrex Laboratories

Vitamin Diagnostics (Pyrrole)

DHA Laboratory (Pyrrole, MSH testing)

European Laboratory of Nutrients (Europe)

Precision Analytical INC. (DUTCH hormone test)

Spectracell Laboratories

Nutritional Resources: Websites

http://www.healthexcel.com

http://bonesandhormones.com/fdn/

http://www.celiac.com

http://www.siboinfo.com

http://thelowhistaminechef.com

http://www.gapsdiet.com

http://paleoleap.com

http://wellnessmama.com

https://www.bulletproofexec.com/61-gluten-sensitivity-celiacs-bulletproofing-your-gut-with-dr-tom-obryan-podcast/

http://whole30.com/whole30-program-rules/

http://www.holistichelp.net/blog/sibo-treatment-diet-and-maintenance/

http://sibodietrecipes.com

http://www.breakingtheviciouscycle.info

http://www.westonaprice.org

http://www.localharvest.org/spring-valley-ny

http://grasslandbeef.com

http://ediblenutmegmagazine.com/about/

http://seafood.edf.org/about-guide

http://www.localharvest.org/new-york-ny

http://www.localharvest.org/farmers-markets/list

http://ohsheglows.com/2013/01/24/my-favourite-homemade-almond-milk-step-by-step-photos/

Find Real Food Locations–Mobile App http://www.findrealfoodapp.com/

http://www.ewg.org/research/ewgs-good-seafood-guide/executive-summary

http://seafood.edf.org/seafood-health-alerts

http://blogs.usda.gov/2012/03/22/organic-101-what-the-usda-organic-label-means/

Wise Choice Market http://www.wisechoicemarket.com/

https://www.ewg.org/foodnews/

Great Lakes Gelatin http://www.greatlakesgelatin.com/

Heritage Foods http://www.heritagefoodsusa.com/

Pure Indian Foods http://www.pureindianfoods.com/

Community Supported Agriculture (CSA)–Just Food http://www.justfood.org/csa

Hawthorn Valley Farm http://hawthornevalleyfarm.org/

http://www.westonaprice.org/health-topics/vegetarianism-and-plant-foods/

http://www.westonaprice.org/health-topics/cod-liver-oil-topics/

http://www.marksdailyapple.com/#axzz4GYQogtH4

Further Reading

Nourishing Traditions: The Cookbook that Challenges Politically Correct Nutrition and Diet Dictocrats by Sally Fallon and Mary G. Enig

Breaking the Vicious Cycle: Intestinal Health Through Diet by Elaine Gloria Gottschall

Know Your Fats: The Complete Primer for Understanding the Nutrition of Fats, Oils, and Cholesterol by Dr. Mary G. Enig

The Fourfold Path to Healing: Working with the Laws of Nutrition, Therapeutics, Movement, and Meditation in the Art of Medicine by Dr. Thomas S. Cowan with Sally Fallon and Jaimen McMillan

Nourishing Traditions Book of Baby and Child Care by Sally Fallon and Tom Cowan, MD

The Gut and Psychology Syndrome by Dr. Natasha Cambell-McBride

The Metabolic Typing Diet: Customize Your Diet to Free Yourself from Food Cravings: Achieve Your Ideal Weight; Enjoy High Energy and Robust Health; Prevent and Reverse Disease by William L. Wolcott and Trish Fahey

A Clinical Guide to Blending Liquid Herbs by Kerry Bone MCPP FNHAA FNIMH DipPhyto Bsc(Hons)

Wild Fermentation and *The Art of Fermentation* by Sandor Katz

Full Moon Feast by Jessica Prentice

Feelings Buried Alive Never Die by Karol K. Truman

Daring Greatly: How the Courage to Be Vulnerable Transforms the Way We Live, Love, Parent, and Lead by Brene Brown

Environmental Toxicity Websites

http://www.ewg.org/tapwater/

http://www.ewg.org/release/new-guide-warns-dirty-dozen-food-additives

http://www.ewg.org/enviroblog/2016/07/
today-s-secret-ingredient-traces-toxic-plastic-chemicals

http://www.womensvoices.org

http://www.safecosmetics.org

https://www.youtube.com/watch?v=vVEi5kIsMuw&list=PLE9FDAC1D62BE268C

http://cdn.ewg.org/sites/default/files/EWGCellphoneTips.pdf?_ga=1.100056798.1554004544
.1410191014

http://www.ewg.org/research/dirty-dozen-list-endocrine-disruptors

http://www.greenmedinfo.com/gmi-blogs-popular

http://www.westonaprice.org/environmental-toxins/

About the Author

In 2006, Rika Kathrin Keck, born and raised in South Africa, founded NY Integrated Health, LLC. With a mind-body philosophy, the company integrates the foundational principles of customized nutrition, lifestyle, and physiological stress management, while also considering the impact of environmental toxins, infections, and genetic predispositions.

Her extensive education bridges the gap from clinical nutrition to functional medicine, and as a nutrition and health expert, Rika has established collaborations with like-minded physicians across the United States. She firmly believes in continuing education and attends various health conferences throughout the year, especially those with physicians who are on the forefront of Lyme disease and biotoxin illness.

All illnesses related to chronic Lyme, coinfections, and mold sickness are of special interest, and this is clearly illustrated in her book, *Nourish, Heal, Thrive: A Comprehensive and Holistic Approach to Living with Lyme Disease.* To her clients, Rika is a trusted advocate, who can support their Lyme-treatment protocol, understands medical testing and lab reports, and knows about the collateral damage from long-term antibiotic or medication use.

Rika also specializes in pre-pregnancy nutrition, digestive wellness, and root-cause investigation of symptoms associated with fibromyalgia, chronic fatigue, and various autoimmune diseases. Her clientele includes children and adults who seek nutritional counseling, drug-free health interventions, and supportive treatment protocols during medical procedures and illness. It is for those who want to integrate a holistic approach for long-term wellness.

In her practice, she places great focus on the initial intake forms, medical history, objective labs, and clinical findings. With her integrated problem-solving approach, this "non-symptom suppressing philosophy" facilitates long-term healing opportunities for her clients who benefit from improved quality of life.

With her extensive knowledge in physiology, metabolic function, and chronic inflammation, Rika provides a valuable bridge between the physician and the patient. It is her passion, and she feels that many need to know the bigger picture that goes beyond Lyme and mold illnesses—and why they might not get better despite treatment.

As a health, fitness, and wellness expert, Rika engages in the corporate wellness arena. She enjoys public speaking opportunities and interactive workshop presentations where she can share her knowledge with passion, sincerity, and a sense of humor.

Rika is also an invited guest blogger on various health blogs where she shares her expertise on a variety of topics.

Through her own experiences of health challenges, Rika herself is witness to the positive and healing effects of an integrated wellness approach. In her spare time, she enjoys traveling, hiking in nature, and cooking at home. Once in a while, she gets her ballet slippers out of retirement and "courageously" attends a ballet class.

For more information, please contact Rika at Rika@NYIntegratedHealth.com or (646)285-8588.